Colitis-Associated Cancer

Masato Kusunoki
Editor

Colitis-Associated Cancer

Springer

Editor
Masato Kusunoki
Mie University Graduate School of Medicine
Department of Gastrointestinal and Pediatric Surgery
Tsu, Japan

ISBN 978-4-431-55521-6 ISBN 978-4-431-55522-3 (eBook)
DOI 10.1007/978-4-431-55522-3

Library of Congress Control Number: 2015952215

Springer Tokyo Heidelberg New York Dordrecht London

Printed on acid-free paper

Springer Japan KK is part of Springer Science+Business Media (www.springer.com)

Preface

In recent decades, there have been tremendous gains in our understanding of the pathogenesis of inflammatory bowel diseases (IBDs), including both ulcerative colitis (UC) and Crohn's disease (CD). Patients with these diseases have a high risk of developing colorectal cancer (CRC), specifically, colitis-associated cancer (CAC), as the repeated episodes of inflammation act as chronic oncogenic insults to the colonic epithelium. In addition, patients with CD, in which the chronic inflammation also involves the small intestine, are at high risk of developing small-bowel adenocarcinoma.

CAC differs from sporadic CRC, both in its histopathological and genetic characteristics. In IBD, the chronic inflammation leads to the increased turnover of epithelial cells, resulting in both low-grade and high-grade dysplasia, and therefore, over time, CAC. This sequence of tumorigenic events is different to that leading to sporadic CRC, although genetic and epigenetic alterations characterize both. CAC has thus been the focus of detailed investigations regarding protein expression; the roles played by the immune response, cytokines, and oxidant stress; the gut bacterial flora; and several other features that contribute to tumorigenesis in patients with IBD.

Despite the extensive experience that has accumulated over many years of managing IBD patients, the diagnosis and treatment of CAC remain controversial. There is widespread agreement regarding the need for surveillance to improve the probability of the early diagnosis of CAC, which is essential given its rapid progression, the poor prognosis of patients diagnosed at a younger age, and the higher mortality associated with CAC than with sporadic CRC. However, whether surveillance reduces CAC-related mortality is unclear. An additional problem is that, in patients with CD, surveillance colonoscopy is difficult because of the presence of colonic strictures, such that most CD-associated CACs and small-bowel tumors are diagnosed in the advanced stage, which implies a poor prognosis. Moreover, surveillance guidelines differ between countries, and a gold standard with respect to endoscopic devices and sampling (e.g., frequency and location) has yet to be defined. Most clinicians recognize the limitations of random biopsy based on its low yield in detecting neoplasia. Instead, chromoendoscopy with targeted biopsies has gained acceptance, and newer endoscopic techniques are being evaluated.

Important advances have been made in the treatment of IBD, although curative treatments remain elusive. In patients with newly detected CAC, surgery, ranging from endoscopic resection to abdominoperineal resection and total proctocolectomy, is the definitive therapeutic approach. However, both the indications for endoscopic treatment and whether the therapeutic benefits of chemotherapy and radiation therapy are the same in CAC as in sporadic CRC are matters of debate. A recent area of investigation is a chemopreventative approach aimed at reducing the inflammation in IBD and thereby also the risk of CAC. Thus, probiotics, immune modulators, and other anti-inflammatory agents are currently being tested.

Basic research into the pathophysiology of IBD has included genome-wide association analysis and the identification of susceptibility genes. These findings have the potential to change clinical practice, predict the natural history of the disease in a particular patient, and guide the choice of therapy. Epigenetics; novel, potentially diagnostic biomarkers; and prognostic markers for CAC have been identified. Molecular alterations in the non-neoplastic mucosa of UC patients, so-called field effects, are promising biomarkers that allow the identification of patients at high risk of CAC. Based on the differential patterns of these markers, it may be possible to predict the progression to carcinogenesis and the responsiveness to therapy. This will give rise to new, patient-tailored therapeutic approaches and more objective surgical indications.

This book provides both an overview of the results of the latest studies on IBD and a summary of the knowledge we have gained through our own experience. It is our hope that, through its brief but informative chapters, readers will acquire a deeper understanding of CAC.

Tsu, Japan M. Kusunoki

Contents

Chapter 1
Colitis-Associated Cancer: Overview

Masato Kusunoki

Abstract In this book, we discuss the pathogenesis and management of colitis-associated colorectal cancer (CAC), including its incidence, risk factors, and prognosis, the genetic alterations leading to tumorigenesis, disease prevention and surveillance options, and medical and surgical treatments.

Among patients with inflammatory bowel diseases (IBD), including ulcerative colitis (UC) and Crohn's disease (CD), CAC is one of the most important causes of mortality. The first reports of CAC (Crohn and Rosenberg. Am J Med Sci 170:220–228, 1925; Warren and Sommers. Gut 48(4):526–535, 2001) showed that its biology and underlying mechanisms distinguish it from sporadic colorectal cancer (CRC). Thus, many different aspects of CAC, such as the histopathological, genetic features, protein expression, the role of the immune response, cytokine disorders, and oxidant stress, and the gut bacterial flora of these patients have been the focus of numerous investigations. Together, they have provided a comprehensive description of the development of CAC.

Keywords Ulcerative colitis • Colorectal cancer • Dysplasia • Diagnosis • Treatment

1.1 Characteristics of CAC in UC

The increased risk of the development of UC-associated CAC (UC-CAC) [1, 2] has been attributed to both genetic and acquired factors. Among the risk factors for developing UC-CAC are the duration [3–5], extent [3, 4, 6–9], and severity [10–13] of colitis, the presence of postinflammatory polyps (pseudopolyps) [10, 12, 14–16], young age at UC onset [3, 6–8], male gender [7, 9], a family history of sporadic CRC [15, 17], and the coexistence of primary sclerosing cholangitis [4, 18, 19]. However, the most important and well-recognized risk factors for UC-CAC are the duration and extent of colitis.

M. Kusunoki (✉)
Department of Gastrointestinal and Pediatric Surgery, Division of Reparative Medicine, Institute of Life Sciences, Mie University Graduate School of Medicine, 2-174 Edobashi, Tsu, Mie 514-8507, Japan
e-mail: surgery2@clin.medic.mie-u.ac.jp

M. Kusunoki (ed.), *Colitis-Associated Cancer*, DOI 10.1007/978-4-431-55522-3_1

UC-CAC shows a more proximal distribution in the colon than CRC, has a higher frequency of multiple synchronous colorectal tumors, and exhibits more aggressive growth and early metastases [20]. CAC tends to be distributed in several locations and to be of higher histologic grade than sporadic cancer [21]. However, according to a report examining each cancer stage, there is no significant difference in the prognosis of CAC vs. sporadic CRC [21–23]. Nonetheless, in the former there is a higher prevalence of mucinous carcinomas [21, 24, 25], which have a relatively worse prognosis than other histologic types of colorectal cancers.

1.2 Role of Endoscopy in UC-CAC

Although recent technical progress in gastroenterological endoscopy, it is still difficult to discriminate between the neoplasms of CC-CAC. This remains the case for dysplasia, which can be difficult to distinguish from normal inflamed mucosa especially in a flat lesion. Thus, surveillance colonoscopy is recommended for the earlier detection and improved prognosis of UC-CAC. Surveillance colonoscopy has been standardized and is now broadly recognized in several guidelines as necessary in patients with long-standing colitis (>8–10 years) in whom there is extended pancolitis or left-sided colitis [26–30]. The prognosis of CAC is considered to better in UC patients who have undergone surveillance colonoscopy than in those who have not [31, 32]. However, in recent guidelines, there are some minor variations regarding the timing of initial screening colonoscopy and the surveillance interval, depending on whether risk stratification has been applied [33–36]. The generally recommended method of surveillance colonoscopy is quadrantic biopsies randomly sampled every 10 cm throughout the colon [33–36]. However, because random biopsy has a low detection rate [37], its use is increasingly discouraged; instead there is increasing focus on target biopsies supported by chromoendoscopy or other newer endoscopic techniques [38–40].

For surveillance, chromoendoscopy allows the detection of dysplasia [38, 41, 42]. The borders of the lesion can be sharply defined using indigo carmine dye spraying as the contrast method. Newer endoscopic techniques, including narrowband imaging [43], fluorescence endoscopy [44, 45], optical coherence tomography [46], and confocal endomicroscopy [41, 46, 47], are being explored as tools to aid in the diagnosis of dysplasia in IBD. Narrowband imaging, a form of virtual chromoendoscopy, can provide a clear image of the microvascular structure, but it is not an alternative to chromoendoscopy for the surveillance for dysplasia [48]. In autofluorescence imaging, the purple-colored neoplasia stands out against the greenish background of normal colonic tissue [49, 50]; however, its effectiveness in UC-CAC remains to be determined. Fluorescence endoscopy commonly employs the blue-fluorescent dye 5-aminolevulinic acid as the sensitizer, based on its selective accumulation in malignant and premalignant tissue [51, 94]. Confocal laser endomicroscopy allows for instant in vivo histology during the course of a standard endoscopy and provides an approximately 1000-fold magnification; but limited data are available thus far [41, 47, 49, 52, 53]. Although there are as yet no randomized controlled trials confirming the effectiveness of surveillance colonoscopy, the Research Group of Intractable Inflammatory Bowel Disease of the Ministry of Health, Labour and Welfare of Japan has conducted a randomized controlled study to compare the efficacy of step biopsy and target biopsy [54]. The results of this study will be reported in the near future.

Total colectomy is currently the gold standard for UC-CAC, because the detection of metachronous neoplasia in the remnant colon and rectum after local resection remains challenging. In low-grade dysplasia (LGD), in which the margins can be diagnostically defined, endoscopic resection can provide an accurate histological diagnosis, but it is technically difficult because in UC the inflammation and fibrosis result in a submucosal layer that is substantially thinner than that of healthy individuals. However, adenoma-like masses (ALMs) can be successfully removed in UC patients using standard polypectomy techniques, with little risk of subsequent malignancy on follow-up [55–58]. In these cases, accurate pathological diagnosis is very important in distinguishing between an ALM and a dysplasia-associated lesion or mass (DALM).

In general, it is often difficult to histologically distinguish dysplasia from non-dysplasia, even by an expert pathologist. Thus, surveillance colonoscopy should be performed during remission phases, which increases the accuracy of histological diagnosis. This is particularly important with respect to the endoscopic resectability of a lesion and in determining its extent; the latter takes precedence over deciding whether the lesion is an ALM or a DALM [5].

1.3 Characteristics of CD-Associated Cancer

The risk of CRC in long-standing CD involving the colon is the same as that in UC [59–62] although the prevalence of CD-associated cancer (CD-CAC) has been increasing. Although the prognosis of CD-CAC is unclear and a wide range of relative risk estimates have been published [63], most reports on the incidence of CD-CAC have been based on patients with a more advanced stage of disease and lymph node involvement than was the case in studies of UC-CAC or non-IBD-related CRC [33, 64–67]. Moreover, CD is associated with a significantly increased risk of small bowel cancer (SBC) [68–71], although it occurs in $<1\ \%$ of CD patients [72, 73]. Nonetheless, the prognosis of cancer, and especially of SBC, against a background of CD is poor because early detection is difficult because of the absence of characteristic symptoms and the difficulty in differentiating malignant disease from CD-related symptoms [74, 75]. In addition, the presence of severe, chronic, complicated, perianal disease in patients with CD seems to be associated with an increased risk of cancer in the anal canal. Carcinoma arising from a perianal fistula, especially a long-standing one, occurs more frequently in patients with CD than in the healthy population [68, 76–81].

1.4 Detection of CAC and SBC in CD

Cancer surveillance programs are thought to reduce the death rate from CD-CAC in patients with colonic disease [82, 83], but there are few data supporting their effectiveness. Moreover, cancer surveillance is often difficult in patients with CD, regardless of the anatomical location of the cancer, because examinations may be limited by the presence of colonic stricture. Thus, up to one-third of patients with IBD develop CAC prior to the initial surveillance [65–67]. Surveillance colonoscopy in patients with CD involving the colon is recommended to assess disease extent and other endoscopic risk factors at least 8–10 years after the onset of disease symptoms [33, 64, 84]. Screening colonoscopy is also recommended in patients with CD colitis involving at least one-third of the length of the colon [35, 84]. The screening interval is based on the estimated risk and on disease duration beginning with the onset of symptoms [33, 84].

The early detection of SBC in patients with CD also remains challenging. A screening and surveillance program for SBC has yet to be established. Routine magnetic resonance enteroclysis/enterography or capsule endoscopy may allow detection of these malignancies at an early stage. However, whether the routine use of these techniques in the screening of asymptomatic individuals can prolong the survival of patients with CD is unclear. Moreover, given the high costs of these procedures, their use remains controversial.

Symptoms in patients with cancer arising from perineal fistulas in CD are usually nonspecific. Consequently, there are no formal guidelines for the screening and surveillance of cancers associated with CD in the lower rectum and perianal region. Carcinoma arising in a CD fistula can be very difficult to diagnose, because the examination for anorectal lesions may be limited by pain, stricture, or induration of the perianal and perineal tissues [80, 85]. Imaging studies, including computed tomography, magnetic resonance imaging (MRI), and 18-fluorodeoxyglucose positron emission tomography (FDG-PET), have a low sensitivity for detecting cancer [80, 85]. Therefore, a high degree of suspicion for carcinoma must be considered in a patient with CD undergoing a rectal examination under anesthesia. The recommended techniques include biopsy, curettage, and brushing of the fistulous tract [86].

1.5 Prevention of CAC

Because chronic inflammation of the large bowel is an important factor for the development of CAC, recent studies have recognized the long-term failure to achieve remission from active colitis as a risk factor [12, 21]. Accordingly, the use of anti-inflammatory agents as chemopreventive agents has been considered. In fact, the most common maintenance therapy in patients with IBD is 5-aminosalicylate. However, while a meta-analysis initially revealed its protective effect with respect to CAC [87], this was not confirmed in subsequent investigations [13, 88–90]. The discrepancy has yet to be resolved. Data on the potential chemopreventive effect of thiopurines in IBD are likewise conflicting [17, 65, 91–93].

Recent data from experimental colitis models have indicated that TNF-α has a tumor-promoting effect [94], and the effect of antibodies targeting tumor necrosis factor (TNF)-α has therefore been evaluated. In a case-control study, anti-TNF-α was shown to protect against the development of CAC [16]. However, most of the studies on chemoprevention in CAC have been retrospective, and various biases have affected their results. This is especially the case when more than one medication was administered for IBD. Thus, whether chemopreventive agents have a role to play in reducing the occurrence of CAC in IBD patients is still unclear.

1.6 Molecular Pathways for CAC

The early detection of IBD-related cancer requires an understanding of the molecular pathways of IBD itself. As noted above, CAC exhibits obvious differences from sporadic CRC with regard to tumor biology. Epithelial cells are sensitive to the balance between pro-and anti-tumorigenic immune factors during inflammation. While colonic inflammation is associated with various tumorigenic events in CAC, their sequence is quite different from those that contribute to the development of sporadic CRC. Development of the latter is characterized as the adenoma → carcinoma sequence, which involves the stepwise accumulation of genetic abnormalities [95]. CAC, however, evolves from LGD to high-grade dysplasia (HGD) to carcinoma and involves multiple genetic alterations. In this process, the inflammatory condition, which consists of an increase in cytokines, chemokines, and reactive oxygen and nitrogen species (RONS), induces DNA mutations, epigenetic alterations, and genomic instability, all of which are well known to be associated with tumor initiation, promotion, and spread [96, 97]. Nonetheless, the molecular mechanisms by which chronic inflammation promotes cancer progression have yet to be fully elucidated.

As noted above, TNF-α is important in cancer development because it acts as a tumor initiator, by stimulating the production of molecules such as those that mediate oxidative stress [98–101]. TNF-α is upregulated in the blood and colonic mucosa of patients with IBD. In an in vivo study of a mouse model of colitis, the use of an anti-TNF-α monoclonal antibody reduced tumor development [97, 102]. Interleukin (IL)-6 is also important in CAC because it promotes the survival of neoplastic colonic epithelial cells [103–108]. The anti-inflammatory cytokine IL-10 downregulates TNF- α, vascular endothelial growth factor, and IL-6 production, which may also account for its inhibitory effect on the tumor stroma [109]. These observations demonstrate a role for the incorrect balance of both pro- and anti-inflammatory cytokines in inflammation and in inflammation-associated carcinogenesis. In fact, animal models have shown that the multifunctional transcription factor nuclear factor B (NF-kB) is required for colorectal neoplasia

[110]. Intraluminal bacterial endotoxins and pro-inflammatory cytokines act through extracellular receptors, such as Toll-like receptors (TLR), to initiate phosphorylation cascades that transmit signals to NF-kB [111, 112]. For example, TLR-4 is upregulated both in UC-CAC and in a mouse model of colon tumors [113].

Oxidative stress caused by the chronic inflammation characteristic of IBD increases the risk of colonic carcinogenesis [114] by inducing nitric oxide synthase, RONS, and free radicals [115–117]. It is also thought that oxidative stress disables the mismatch repair system and thereby causes genomic instability [118, 119]. Genomic instability can be divided into two clinically distinct forms that have been extensively studied in CRC: chromosomal instability (CIN) and microsatellite instability (MSI) [120].

CIN is typically associated with the progressive accumulation of mutations in onco-suppressor genes, such as the adenomatous polyposis coli (APC) and p53 genes, and oncogenes such as KRAS. Loss of APC function is a very common initiating event in sporadic CRC, but it is less frequent and usually occurs later in CAC [121–124]. Mutations in p53 are part of the early process of tumorigenesis, i.e., in preneoplastic lesions or those indefinite for dysplasia [125–127]. The loss of p53 function, observed in over half of the cases of CAC, is an important step in disease progression [125, 127, 128]. Conversely, the KRAS mutation plays a significant role in the later stage of CAC, as is the case in sporadic CRC [129], but its detection rate is lower in the former [130, 131].

MSI reflects alterations in or the inactivation of DNA repair mechanisms, including nucleotide excision repair, base excision repair, and mismatch repair [132]. An association of UC-CAC with MSI has been demonstrated, and the high rate of MSI in long-standing UC is probably related to the genomic instability produced by repeated inflammatory stimulations [133].

For both CIN and MSI, epigenetic elements can affect tumor initiation, proliferation, and metastasis in CAC. For example, the hypermethylation of onco-suppressor DNA promoter regions and microRNAs are two major epigenetic mechanisms of gene silencing that are involved in the development and progression of colorectal carcinogenesis [134]. Epigenetic alterations are also observed during inflammation and inflammation-associated carcinogenesis [135, 136]. The methylation of CpG islands in several genes precedes dysplasia and can be detected throughout the mucosa of patients with UC [137]. A significant relationship between DNA methylation and MSI in UC patients has been reported [138, 139]. Therefore, the inactivation of promoter hypermethylation may be critical in preventing the accumulation of inflamed, genetically damaged epithelial cells in UC and thus for preventing the initiation of the carcinogenetic process and the development of CAC. Inflammation-induced DNA methylation is related to oxidative stress and increased levels of pro-inflammatory cytokines [108, 140–142]. The mechanisms of how these pro-inflammatory mediators alter the DNA methylation pattern during inflammation are not completely understood, but in a mouse model of colitis, aberrant DNA methylation was detected even in the absence of macroscopic tumors and gradually increased until they developed

[143]. Therefore, the duration of inflammation is an important factor in aberrant DNA methylation, which is consistent with the duration of IBD being a risk factor for the development of CAC.

A role for microRNA (miRNA) has also been described. miRNA acts posttranscriptionally and is one of the major regulators of gene expression [144] during cellular differentiation, development, proliferation, and apoptosis. It also contributes to the initiation and progression of cancer in carcinogenesis [145]. In general, the expression profiles of tumor-specific miRNAs are more informative and discriminatory than mRNA profiles. Furthermore, circulating miRNAs are highly resistant to RNase activity, unlike mRNA [146]. There are reports showing higher miRNA levels in IBD-associated dysplastic lesions than in active IBD [147] and that the levels increase successively at each stage of IBD progression [148, 149]. However, miRNA-based markers for identifying UC patients who are at increased risk of neoplasia are still at the early stage of development, as described in the following section.

1.7 Molecular Markers for Identifying CAC

An improved prognosis of patients with CAC requires diagnosis of the disease at an early or precancerous stage and therefore more accurate diagnostic modalities, such as the analysis of p53 alterations for distinguishing neoplastic lesions from regenerative epithelium. The molecular alterations in gene expression and in the form of CIN, MSI, DNA aneuploidy, DNA methylation, and telomere shortening in nonneoplastic UC mucosa, so-called field effects, are being explored as promising biomarkers for use in identifying UC patients at high risk of CAC. In addition, because age-related methylation may be an important contributor to the acquired predisposition to colorectal neoplasia, it may serve as a molecular marker in this population [137, 150, 151].

1.8 Surgical Indications for UC-CAC

In UC patients, the detection of CAC on biopsy is an absolute indication for surgery. However, the decision-making process in patients with UC who, after a diagnosis of dysplasia, are considering intensive surveillance rather than surgical intervention is a difficult one. The detection of HGD is an absolute indication for surgical resection regardless of previous surgical treatment [25, 152]. Moreover, as noted above, any DALM, in particular one associated with a polypoid mass, indicates a high likelihood of the presence of synchronous or metachronous neoplasia, considered to be endoscopically unresectable [153]. Thus, patients with UC who are diagnosed with non-adenoma-like DALMs, regardless of the dysplasia grade detected on biopsy, should undergo colectomy [35, 153, 154]. Indeed, advanced neoplasia can be found in association with dysplastic changes of any grade [155, 156]. However, the strategy for patients with LGD varies slightly according to the guidelines [35, 36, 64]. Although controversial, there is evidence to suggest that patients with flat, unifocal LGD should consider colectomy [28, 84].

Surgical procedures for neoplasia in patients with UC range from colonoscopic resection to total proctocolectomy (TPC). The choice of surgical treatment is influenced by the site and stage of the cancer, the functional state of the rectum, the presence of multifocal lesions, the patient's age, and the duration of UC [157]. Abdominoperineal TPC is the definitive treatment for the eradication of undiagnosed synchronous dysplasias and/or carcinomas and the prevention of subsequent metachronous lesions in UC; therefore, it is the only operation that will reliably eliminate the cancer risk in UC. However, this procedure requires permanent ileostomy, such that it is indicated mostly in patients with advanced-stage cancer of the rectum and anal canal and in patients with poor anal sphincter function, such as the older postpartum female.

The efficacy of segmental colectomy in patients with UC in long-term remission is a matter of debate. Generally, segmental resection of the colon should be avoided for CAC because of the high frequency of occult carcinomas and multifocal carcinogenesis, such that a residual lesion and therefore postoperative relapse is not rare [158]. If the colitis is totally quiescent or exhibits rectal sparing, total abdominal colectomy with ileorectal anastomosis (IRA) may be recommended as an option for UC patients with a single cancer in the colon. Low anterior resection (LAR) should be considered very carefully in patients with quiescent UC and rectal cancer or dysplasia because further proctocolectomy and IPAA would be difficult after LAR. In addition, a relapse of inflammation in the residual rectum must be taken into account. Subtotal colectomy with end ileostomy and a rectal stump pouch are less ideal options because of the retained rectum, which represents a continued cancer risk. While this procedure has previously been demonstrated as a safe treatment option, some of these patients will be satisfied with an ileostomy. Others may not be eligible because of their comorbidities and will refuse later pelvic pouch surgery.

1.9 TPC with IPAA for UC-CAC

The gold standard procedure for patients with UC is TPC with IPAA. Whether with or without mucosal proctectomy (stapled or hand-sewn IPAAs), these procedures are indicated for any colonic or rectal neoplasms in the surgically fit patient. However, controversy remains regarding these two procedures in UC-CAC because of the risk that the patient will later develop synchronous or metachronous neoplasias in the retained anal transitional zone (ATZ) mucosa. If stapled IPAA is performed, both long-term surveillance to monitor dysplasia and repeat biopsies from the remnant ATZ are required. Clearly, the presence of dysplasia in the ATZ is a contraindication for stapled IPAA. Moreover, hand-sewn IPAA is strongly recommended especially for cancers or HGD outside the ATZ because the incidence of dysplasia after stapled IPAA is not trivial [124, 159–166]. By contrast, there have been several reports of cancer occurrence from the residual ATZ even after hand-sewn IPAA with mucosectomy [159, 167]. Thus, routine long-term endoscopic surveillance is recommended in patients with long-standing ileal pouches even after mucosectomy of the ATZ and especially in the presence of dysplasia or cancer in the proctocolectomy specimen.

1.10 Prognosis After Surgery for UC-CAC

The survival of patients with UC-CAC is slightly poorer than that of patients with sporadic CRC; however, the detection of UC-CAC at an early stage results in the similar survival of the two groups [21, 22] For locally advanced rectal cancer in patients with UC, multimodality therapies such as chemotherapy and radiotherapy are required. Whether preoperative chemoradiotherapy reduces the incidence of postoperative complications is controversial [166, 168, 169]. The prognosis after surgery for UC-CAC depends on the presence of neoplasia in the ileal pouch and the overall outcome. Although the cumulative incidence of neoplasia involving the ileal pouch is very low, a history of colorectal neoplasia and chronic inflammation of the ileal mucosa, such as preoperative backwash ileitis, and postoperative pouchitis are risk factors associated with pouch neoplasia [170–175]. It is therefore recommended that patients with these risk factors be followed by endoscopy and random biopsies for the rest of their lives.

1.11 Treatment of CAC and SBC in CD

In the surgical treatment of cancer associated with CD, the malignancy should be diagnosed with respect to its location, i.e., small intestinal, colonic, or anorectal. Because SBC is less frequent and is difficult to detect prior to surgery, its final diagnosis is often made based on perioperative or postoperative pathological examination results [176]. For CD-associated cancers in general, although their early-stage detection is challenging, FDG-PET has shown promise in the assessment of these tumors [177]. The objective of surgery for cancer in CD is resection for cure or, when indicated, palliation and the removal of associated or discontinuous segments of inflammatory disease.

Segmental resection is the surgical approach for treating SBC in segmental CD. In patients with multiple strictures of the small bowel, concomitant strictureplasties should be performed in addition to resection of the malignant stricture. Prior to strictureplasty, each stricture should be biopsied, with the evaluation of frozen sections, to rule out the presence of synchronous cancers. Segmental resection is also the surgical procedure of choice for colonic cancer in segmental

CD. However, subtotal colectomy is chosen in patients with CD of the colon with malignant degeneration but rectal sparing.

TPC is generally performed for patients with CAC and pancolitis or with segmental colonic and rectal disease or with colonic and severe perianal disease. Whether TPC is required for colorectal cancer or dysplasia in CD, as is the case in UC, or whether segmental resection might be adequate remains controversial [178]. In CD, once dysplasia is identified, segmental resection is a more feasible option, especially if there has been a consistent lack of inflammation elsewhere in the intestinal tract [178]. By contrast, TPC should be performed in patients with multifocal colonic dysplasia or rectal dysplasia.

Cancer involving an internal or external fistula and occurring in combination with an intestinal lesion of CD is uncommon. In these cases, the early-stage detection of the disease is very difficult, such that most of these tumors are unresectable. Occasionally, however, a radical en bloc resection that includes the fistula is possible.

In CD, anal cancers are more often adenocarcinoma than squamous cell carcinoma. Mucinous adenocarcinoma, a more aggressive type of CRC [179], occurs in approximately 50 % of CD-CAC cases. The prognosis of cancer associated with anorectal lesions is poor, although some reports have suggested that it can be improved by preoperative chemoradiotherapy. There is no evidence regarding the efficacy of adjuvant chemoradiation in CD patients with anorectal adenocarcinoma. In fact, mucinous anorectal adenocarcinoma seems to respond poorly to chemoradiation [180–182].

In the great majority of patients, the surgical treatment of rectal and anal cancers associated with CD involves proctectomy. In addition, the colon should be resected or totally removed depending on the extent of the inflammation [77]. Treatment can be curative if the diagnosis is made early. Since rectal amputation is unavoidable for most patients with cancer associated with anorectal lesions, abdominoperineal resection is the most frequently employed procedure [183–185].

Postoperative complications often occur after surgery for anorectal cancer associated with CD. Among these, perineal wound infection may result in a persistent perineal sinus. The management strategy for perineal wound problems will depend on the patient's condition and the surgeon's preference. Great care is necessary intraoperatively, as postoperative sexual and urinary dysfunction often result from intraoperative autonomic nerve injury.

There are no data on the value and benefit of adjuvant therapy after curative resection of gastrointestinal cancers in CD. For the occasional patient with cancer complicating CD, the same recommendations for adjuvant therapy in sporadic CRC patients undergoing resection can be adopted.

References

1. Crohn B, Rosenberg H (1925) The sigmoidoscopic picture of chronic ulcerative colitis (non-specific). Am J Med Sci 170:220–228
2. Warren S, Sommers SC (1948) Cicatrizing enteritis as a pathologic entity; analysis of 120 cases. Am J Pathol 24(3):475–501
3. Eaden JA, Abrams KR, Mayberry JF (2001) The risk of colorectal cancer in ulcerative colitis: a meta-analysis. Gut 48(4):526–535
4. Lakatos L et al (2006) Risk factors for ulcerative colitis-associated colorectal cancer in a Hungarian cohort of patients with ulcerative colitis: results of a population-based study. Inflamm Bowel Dis 12(3):205–211
5. Rutter MD et al (2006) Thirty-year analysis of a colonoscopic surveillance program for neoplasia in ulcerative colitis. Gastroenterology 130(4):1030–1038
6. Lutgens MW et al (2013) Declining risk of colorectal cancer in inflammatory bowel disease: an updated meta-analysis of population-based cohort studies. Inflamm Bowel Dis 19 (4):789–799
7. Jess T, Rungoe C, Peyrin-Biroulet L (2012) Risk of colorectal cancer in patients with ulcerative colitis: a meta-analysis of population-based cohort studies. Clin Gastroenterol Hepatol 10(6):639–645
8. Ekbom A et al (1990) Ulcerative colitis and colorectal cancer. A population-based study. N Engl J Med 323(18):1228–1233
9. Soderlund S et al (2009) Decreasing time-trends of colorectal cancer in a large cohort of patients with inflammatory bowel disease. Gastroenterology 136(5):1561–1567, quiz 1818–9
10. Rutter MD et al (2004) Cancer surveillance in longstanding ulcerative colitis: endoscopic appearances help predict cancer risk. Gut 53(12):1813–1816
11. Gupta RB et al (2007) Histologic inflammation is a risk factor for progression to colorectal neoplasia in ulcerative colitis: a cohort study. Gastroenterology 133(4):1099–1105, quiz 1340–1
12. Rutter M et al (2004) Severity of inflammation is a risk factor for colorectal neoplasia in ulcerative colitis. Gastroenterology 126(2):451–459
13. Jess T et al (2007) Risk factors for colorectal neoplasia in inflammatory bowel disease: a nested case-control study from Copenhagen county, Denmark and Olmsted county, Minnesota. Am J Gastroenterol 102(4):829–836
14. Lovasz BD et al (2013) Risk of colorectal cancer in Crohn's disease patients with colonic involvement and stenosing disease in a population-based cohort from Hungary. J Gastrointestin Liver Dis 22(3):265–268
15. Velayos FS et al (2006) Predictive and protective factors associated with colorectal cancer in ulcerative colitis: A case-control study. Gastroenterology 130(7):1941–1949
16. Baars JE et al (2011) The risk of inflammatory bowel disease-related colorectal carcinoma is limited: results from a nationwide nested case-control study. Am J Gastroenterol 106 (2):319–328
17. Askling J et al (2001) Family history as a risk factor for colorectal cancer in inflammatory bowel disease. Gastroenterology 120(6):1356–1362
18. Broome U, Lindberg G, Lofberg R (1992) Primary sclerosing cholangitis in ulcerative colitis–a risk factor for the development of dysplasia and DNA aneuploidy? Gastroenterology 102(6):1877–1880
19. Soetikno RM et al (2002) Increased risk of colorectal neoplasia in patients with primary sclerosing cholangitis and ulcerative colitis: a meta-analysis. Gastrointest Endosc 56 (1):48–54
20. Ren LL, Fang JY (2011) Should we sound the alarm? Dysplasia and colitis-associated colorectal cancer. Asian Pac J Cancer Prev 12(8):1881–1886
21. Delaunoit T et al (2006) Colorectal cancer prognosis among patients with inflammatory bowel disease. Clin Gastroenterol Hepatol 4(3):335–342

22. Watanabe T et al (2011) Ulcerative colitis-associated colorectal cancer shows a poorer survival than sporadic colorectal cancer: a nationwide Japanese study. Inflamm Bowel Dis 17(3):802–808
23. Lavery IC et al (1982) Survival with carcinoma arising in mucosal ulcerative colitis. Ann Surg 195(4):508–512
24. Fogt F et al (1998) Comparison of genetic alterations in colonic adenoma and ulcerative colitis-associated dysplasia and carcinoma. Hum Pathol 29(2):131–136
25. Nugent FW et al (1979) Malignant potential of chronic ulcerative colitis. Preliminary report. Gastroenterology 76(1):1–5
26. Kornbluth A, Sachar DB (1997) Ulcerative colitis practice guidelines in adults. American College of Gastroenterology, Practice Parameters Committee. Am J Gastroenterol 92 (2):204–211
27. Leighton JA et al (2006) ASGE guideline: endoscopy in the diagnosis and treatment of inflammatory bowel disease. Gastrointest Endosc 63(4):558–565
28. Eaden JA, Mayberry JF (2002) Guidelines for screening and surveillance of asymptomatic colorectal cancer in patients with inflammatory bowel disease. Gut 51(Suppl 5):V10–V12
29. Ooi CJ et al (2010) The Asia-Pacific consensus on ulcerative colitis. J Gastroenterol Hepatol 25(3):453–468
30. Hida N et al (2014) A questionnaire-based survey on the diagnosis and management of inflammatory bowel disease in East Asian countries in 2012. Digestion 89(1):88–103
31. Choi PM et al (1993) Colonoscopic surveillance reduces mortality from colorectal cancer in ulcerative colitis. Gastroenterology 105(2):418–424
32. Connell WR et al (1994) Factors affecting the outcome of endoscopic surveillance for cancer in ulcerative colitis. Gastroenterology 107(4):934–944
33. Cairns SR et al (2010) Guidelines for colorectal cancer screening and surveillance in moderate and high risk groups (update from 2002). Gut 59(5):666–689
34. Van Assche G et al (2013) Second European evidence-based consensus on the diagnosis and management of ulcerative colitis part 3: special situations. J Crohns Colitis 7(1):1–33
35. Farraye FA et al (2010) AGA technical review on the diagnosis and management of colorectal neoplasia in inflammatory bowel disease. Gastroenterology 138(2):746–774, 774 e1-4; quiz e12-3
36. Kornbluth A, Sachar DB (2010) Ulcerative colitis practice guidelines in adults: American College Of Gastroenterology, Practice Parameters Committee. Am J Gastroenterol 105 (3):501–523, quiz 524
37. van den Broek FJ et al (2014) Random biopsies taken during colonoscopic surveillance of patients with longstanding ulcerative colitis: low yield and absence of clinical consequences. Am J Gastroenterol 109(5):715–722
38. Rutter MD et al (2004) Pancolonic indigo carmine dye spraying for the detection of dysplasia in ulcerative colitis. Gut 53(2):256–260
39. Hurlstone DP et al (2008) Confocal chromoscopic endomicroscopy is superior to chromoscopy alone for the detection and characterisation of intraepithelial neoplasia in chronic ulcerative colitis. Gut 57(2):196–204
40. Hurlstone DP et al (2005) Indigo carmine-assisted high-magnification chromoscopic colonoscopy for the detection and characterisation of intraepithelial neoplasia in ulcerative colitis: a prospective evaluation. Endoscopy 37(12):1186–1192
41. Kiesslich R et al (2007) Chromoscopy-guided endomicroscopy increases the diagnostic yield of intraepithelial neoplasia in ulcerative colitis. Gastroenterology 132(3):874–882
42. Marion JF et al (2008) Chromoendoscopy-targeted biopsies are superior to standard colonoscopic surveillance for detecting dysplasia in inflammatory bowel disease patients: a prospective endoscopic trial. Am J Gastroenterol 103(9):2342–2349
43. Dekker E et al (2007) Narrow-band imaging compared with conventional colonoscopy for the detection of dysplasia in patients with longstanding ulcerative colitis. Endoscopy 39 (3):216–221

44. Matsumoto T et al (2007) Autofluorescence imaging colonoscopy for the diagnosis of dysplasia in ulcerative colitis. Inflamm Bowel Dis 13(5):640–641
45. Messmann H et al (2003) Fluorescence endoscopy for the detection of low and high grade dysplasia in ulcerative colitis using systemic or local 5-aminolaevulinic acid sensitisation. Gut 52(7):1003–1007
46. Kiesslich R, Neurath MF (2008) What new endoscopic imaging modalities will become important in the diagnosis of IBD? Inflamm Bowel Dis 14(Suppl 2):S172–S176
47. Kiesslich R et al (2004) Confocal laser endoscopy for diagnosing intraepithelial neoplasias and colorectal cancer in vivo. Gastroenterology 127(3):706–713
48. Efthymiou M et al (2013) Chromoendoscopy versus narrow band imaging for colonic surveillance in inflammatory bowel disease. Inflamm Bowel Dis 19(10):2132–2138
49. Bessissow T, Bisschops R (2013) Advanced endoscopic imaging for dysplasia surveillance in ulcerative colitis. Expert Rev Gastroenterol Hepatol 7(1):57–67
50. van den Broek FJ et al (2008) Endoscopic tri-modal imaging for surveillance in ulcerative colitis: randomised comparison of high-resolution endoscopy and autofluorescence imaging for neoplasia detection; and evaluation of narrow-band imaging for classification of lesions. Gut 57(8):1083–1089
51. Peng Q et al (1997) 5-Aminolevulinic acid-based photodynamic therapy. Clinical research and future challenges. Cancer 79(12):2282–2308
52. Guagnozzi D, Lucendo AJ (2012) Colorectal cancer surveillance in patients with inflammatory bowel disease: What is new? World J Gastrointest Endosc 4(4):108–116
53. Neumann H et al (2010) Confocal laser endomicroscopy: technical advances and clinical applications. Gastroenterology 139(2):388–392, 392 e1-2
54. Watanabe T et al (2011) Target biopsy or step biopsy? Optimal surveillance for ulcerative colitis: a Japanese nationwide randomized controlled trial. J Gastroenterol 46(Suppl 1):11–16
55. Odze RD et al (2004) Long-term follow-up after polypectomy treatment for adenoma-like dysplastic lesions in ulcerative colitis. Clin Gastroenterol Hepatol 2(7):534–541
56. Engelsgjerd M, Farraye FA, Odze RD (1999) Polypectomy may be adequate treatment for adenoma-like dysplastic lesions in chronic ulcerative colitis. Gastroenterology 117 (6):1288–1294, discussion 1488–91
57. Monkemuller K et al (2009) Advanced colon polypectomy. Clin Gastroenterol Hepatol 7 (6):641–652
58. Vieth M, Behrens H, Stolte M (2006) Sporadic adenoma in ulcerative colitis: endoscopic resection is an adequate treatment. Gut 55(8):1151–1155
59. Softley A et al (1988) The natural history of inflammatory bowel disease: has there been a change in the last 20 years? Scand J Gastroenterol Suppl 144:20–23
60. Richards ME, Rickert RR, Nance FC (1989) Crohn's disease-associated carcinoma. A poorly recognized complication of inflammatory bowel disease. Ann Surg 209(6):764–773
61. Stahl TJ et al (1992) Crohn's disease and carcinoma: increasing justification for surveillance? Dis Colon Rectum 35(9):850–856
62. Maykel JA et al (2006) Crohn's colitis: the incidence of dysplasia and adenocarcinoma in surgical patients. Dis Colon Rectum 49(7):950–957
63. Canavan C, Abrams KR, Mayberry J (2006) Meta-analysis: colorectal and small bowel cancer risk in patients with Crohn's disease. Aliment Pharmacol Ther 23(8):1097–1104
64. Farraye FA et al (2010) AGA medical position statement on the diagnosis and management of colorectal neoplasia in inflammatory bowel disease. Gastroenterology 138(2):738–745
65. Beaugerie L et al (2013) Risk of colorectal high-grade dysplasia and cancer in a prospective observational cohort of patients with inflammatory bowel disease. Gastroenterology 145 (1):166–175, e8
66. Jess T et al (2012) Decreasing risk of colorectal cancer in patients with inflammatory bowel disease over 30 years. Gastroenterology 143(2) 375–381, e1; quiz e13-4

67. Baars JE et al (2012) Age at diagnosis of inflammatory bowel disease influences early development of colorectal cancer in inflammatory bowel disease patients: a nationwide, long-term survey. J Gastroenterol 47(12):1308–1322
68. Jess T et al (2005) Increased risk of intestinal cancer in Crohn's disease: a meta-analysis of population-based cohort studies. Am J Gastroenterol 100(12):2724–2729
69. von Roon AC et al (2007) The risk of cancer in patients with Crohn's disease. Dis Colon Rectum 50(6):839–855
70. Laukoetter MG et al (2011) Intestinal cancer risk in Crohn's disease: a meta-analysis. J Gastrointest Surg 15(4):576–583
71. Kamiya T et al (2012) Intestinal cancers occurring in patients with Crohn's disease. J Gastroenterol Hepatol 27(Suppl 3):103–107
72. Michelassi F et al (1993) Adenocarcinoma complicating Crohn's disease. Dis Colon Rectum 36(7):654–661
73. Higashi D et al (2013) Cancer of the small intestine in patients with Crohn's disease. Anticancer Res 33(7):2977–2980
74. Elriz K et al (2013) Incidence, presentation, and prognosis of small bowel adenocarcinoma in patients with small bowel Crohn's disease: a prospective observational study. Inflamm Bowel Dis 19(9):1823–1826
75. Dossett LA et al (2007) Small bowel adenocarcinoma complicating Crohn's disease: case series and review of the literature. Am Surg 73(11):1181–1187
76. Ky A et al (1998) Carcinoma arising in anorectal fistulas of Crohn's disease. Dis Colon Rectum 41(8):992–996
77. Sjodahl RI, Myrelid P, Soderholm JD (2003) Anal and rectal cancer in Crohn's disease. Color Dis 5(5):490–495
78. Connell WR et al (1994) Lower gastrointestinal malignancy in Crohn's disease. Gut 35 (3):347–352
79. Higashi D et al (2007) Study of colorectal cancer with Crohn's disease. Anticancer Res 27 (6A):3771–3774
80. Iesalnieks I et al (2010) Fistula-associated anal adenocarcinoma in Crohn's disease. Inflamm Bowel Dis 16(10):1643–1648
81. Baars JE et al (2011) Malignant transformation of perianal and enterocutaneous fistulas is rare: results of 17 years of follow-up from The Netherlands. Scand J Gastroenterol 46 (3):319–325
82. Mpofu C, Watson AJ, Rhodes JM (2004) Strategies for detecting colon cancer and/or dysplasia in patients with inflammatory bowel disease. Cochrane Database Syst Rev 2: CD000279
83. Collins PD et al (2006) Strategies for detecting colon cancer and/or dysplasia in patients with inflammatory bowel disease. Cochrane Database Syst Rev 2:CD000279
84. Itzkowitz SH et al (2005) Consensus conference: Colorectal cancer screening and surveillance in inflammatory bowel disease. Inflamm Bowel Dis 11(3):314–321
85. Devon KM et al (2009) Cancer of the anus complicating perianal Crohn's disease. Dis Colon Rectum 52(2):211–216
86. Laurent S et al (2005) Development of adenocarcinoma in chronic fistula in Crohn's disease. Acta Gastroenterol Belg 68(1):98–100
87. Velayos FS, Terdiman JP, Walsh JM (2005) Effect of 5-aminosalicylate use on colorectal cancer and dysplasia risk: a systematic review and metaanalysis of observational studies. Am J Gastroenterol 100(6):1345–1353
88. Bernstein CN, Nugent Z, Blanchard JF (2011) 5-aminosalicylate is not chemoprophylactic for colorectal cancer in IBD: a population based study. Am J Gastroenterol 106(4):731–736
89. Terdiman JP et al (2007) 5-Aminosalicylic acid therapy and the risk of colorectal cancer among patients with inflammatory bowel disease. Inflamm Bowel Dis 13(4):367–371

90. Nguyen GC, Gulamhusein A, Bernstein CN (2012) 5-aminosalicylic acid is not protective against colorectal cancer in inflammatory bowel disease: a meta-analysis of non-referral populations. Am J Gastroenterol 107(9):1298–1304, quiz 1297, 1305
91. van Schaik FD et al (2012) Thiopurines prevent advanced colorectal neoplasia in patients with inflammatory bowel disease. Gut 61(2):235–240
92. Pasternak B et al (2013) Use of azathioprine and the risk of cancer in inflammatory bowel disease. Am J Epidemiol 177(11):1296–1305
93. Armstrong RG, West J, Card TR (2010) Risk of cancer in inflammatory bowel disease treated with azathioprine: a UK population-based case-control study. Am J Gastroenterol 105 (7):1604–1609
94. Onizawa M et al (2009) Signaling pathway via TNF-alpha/NF-kappaB in intestinal epithelial cells may be directly involved in colitis-associated carcinogenesis. Am J Physiol Gastrointest Liver Physiol 296(4):G850–G859
95. Fearon ER, Vogelstein B (1990) A genetic model for colorectal tumorigenesis. Cell 61 (5):759–767
96. Karin M, Greten FR (2005) NF-kappaB: linking inflammation and immunity to cancer development and progression. Nat Rev Immunol 5(10):749–759
97. Grivennikov SI, Greten FR, Karin M (2010) Immunity, inflammation, and cancer. Cell 140 (6):883–899
98. Noguchi M et al (1998) Secretion imbalance between tumour necrosis factor and its inhibitor in inflammatory bowel disease. Gut 43(2):203–209
99. Wallis RS (2008) Tumour necrosis factor antagonists: structure, function, and tuberculosis risks. Lancet Infect Dis 8(10):601–611
100. Di Girolamo N et al (1997) Expression of TNF-alpha by human plasma cells in chronic inflammation. J Leukoc Biol 61(6):667–678
101. Szlosarek P, Charles KA, Balkwill FR (2006) Tumour necrosis factor-alpha as a tumour promoter. Eur J Cancer 42(6):745–750
102. Popivanova BK et al (2008) Blocking TNF-alpha in mice reduces colorectal carcinogenesis associated with chronic colitis. J Clin Invest 118(2):560–570
103. Bromberg J, Wang TC (2009) Inflammation and cancer: IL-6 and STAT3 complete the link. Cancer Cell 15(2):79–80
104. Bollrath J et al (2009) gp130-mediated Stat3 activation in enterocytes regulates cell survival and cell-cycle progression during colitis-associated tumorigenesis. Cancer Cell 15(2):91–102
105. Esfandi F, Mohammadzadeh Ghobadloo S, Basati G (2006) Interleukin-6 level in patients with colorectal cancer. Cancer Lett 244(1):76–78
106. Li Y et al (2010) Disease-related expression of the IL6/STAT3/SOCS3 signalling pathway in ulcerative colitis and ulcerative colitis-related carcinogenesis. Gut 59(2):227–235
107. Matsumoto S et al (2010) Essential roles of IL-6 trans-signaling in colonic epithelial cells, induced by the IL-6/soluble-IL-6 receptor derived from lamina propria macrophages, on the development of colitis-associated premalignant cancer in a murine model. J Immunol 184 (3):1543–1551
108. Foran E et al (2010) Upregulation of DNA methyltransferase-mediated gene silencing, anchorage-independent growth, and migration of colon cancer cells by interleukin-6. Mol Cancer Res 8(4):471–481
109. Huang S, Ullrich SE, Bar-Eli M (1999) Regulation of tumor growth and metastasis by interleukin-10: the melanoma experience. J Interferon Cytokine Res 19(7):697–703
110. Greten FR et al (2004) IKKbeta links inflammation and tumorigenesis in a mouse model of colitis-associated cancer. Cell 118(3):285–296
111. Fukata M, Abreu MT (2008) Role of Toll-like receptors in gastrointestinal malignancies. Oncogene 27(2):234–243
112. Maeda S, Omata M (2008) Inflammation and cancer: role of nuclear factor-kappaB activation. Cancer Sci 99(5):836–842

113. Fukata M et al (2007) Toll-like receptor-4 promotes the development of colitis-associated colorectal tumors. Gastroenterology 133(6):1869–1881
114. Hussain SP, Hofseth LJ, Harris CC (2003) Radical causes of cancer. Nat Rev Cancer 3 (4):276–285
115. Hofseth LJ et al (2003) Nitric oxide-induced cellular stress and p53 activation in chronic inflammation. Proc Natl Acad Sci U S A 100(1):143–148
116. Kimura H et al (1998) Increased expression of an inducible isoform of nitric oxide synthase and the formation of peroxynitrite in colonic mucosa of patients with active ulcerative colitis. Gut 42(2):180–187
117. Rachmilewitz D et al (1995) Enhanced colonic nitric oxide generation and nitric oxide synthase activity in ulcerative colitis and Crohn's disease. Gut 36(5):718–723
118. Chang CL et al (2002) Oxidative stress inactivates the human DNA mismatch repair system. Am J Physiol Cell Physiol 283(1):C148–C154
119. Brentnall TA et al (1996) Microsatellite instability in nonneoplastic mucosa from patients with chronic ulcerative colitis. Cancer Res 56(6):1237–1240
120. Lengauer C, Kinzler KW, Vogelstein B (1998) Genetic instabilities in human cancers. Nature 396(6712):643–649
121. Aust DE et al (2002) The APC/beta-catenin pathway in ulcerative colitis-related colorectal carcinomas: a mutational analysis. Cancer 94(5):1421–1427
122. Tarmin L et al (1995) Adenomatous polyposis coli gene mutations in ulcerative colitis-associated dysplasias and cancers versus sporadic colon neoplasms. Cancer Res 55 (10):2035–2038
123. Redston MS et al (1995) Common occurrence of APC and K-ras gene mutations in the spectrum of colitis-associated neoplasias. Gastroenterology 108(2):383–392
124. Johnston D et al (1987) Preservation of the entire anal canal in conservative proctocolectomy for ulcerative colitis: a pilot study comparing end-to-end ileo-anal anastomosis without mucosal resection with mucosal proctectomy and endo-anal anastomosis. Br J Surg 74 (10):940–944
125. Burmer GC et al (1992) Neoplastic progression in ulcerative colitis: histology, DNA content, and loss of a p53 allele. Gastroenterology 103(5):1602–1610
126. Brentnall TA et al (1994) Mutations in the p53 gene: an early marker of neoplastic progression in ulcerative colitis. Gastroenterology 107(2):369–378
127. Yin J et al (1993) p53 point mutations in dysplastic and cancerous ulcerative colitis lesions. Gastroenterology 104(6):1633–1639
128. Hussain SP et al (2000) Increased p53 mutation load in noncancerous colon tissue from ulcerative colitis: a cancer-prone chronic inflammatory disease. Cancer Res 60 (13):3333–3337
129. Vogelstein B et al (1988) Genetic alterations during colorectal-tumor development. N Engl J Med 319(9):525–532
130. Benhattar J, Saraga E (1995) Molecular genetics of dysplasia in ulcerative colitis. Eur J Cancer 31A(7–8):1171–1173
131. Andersen SN et al (1999) Villous, hypermucinous mucosa in long standing ulcerative colitis shows high frequency of K-ras mutations. Gut 45(5):686–692
132. Charames GS, Bapat B (2003) Genomic instability and cancer. Curr Mol Med 3(7):589–596
133. Ishitsuka T, Kashiwagi H, Konishi F (2001) Microsatellite instability in inflamed and neoplastic epithelium in ulcerative colitis. J Clin Pathol 54(7):526–532
134. D'Inca R et al (2004) Oxidative DNA damage in the mucosa of ulcerative colitis increases with disease duration and dysplasia. Inflamm Bowel Dis 10(1):23–27
135. Saito S et al (2011) DNA methylation of colon mucosa in ulcerative colitis patients: correlation with inflammatory status. Inflamm Bowel Dis 17(9):1955–1965
136. Glauben R et al (2006) Histone hyperacetylation is associated with amelioration of experimental colitis in mice. J Immunol 176(8):5015–5022

137. Issa JP et al (2001) Accelerated age-related CpG island methylation in ulcerative colitis. Cancer Res 61(9):3573–3577
138. Fleisher AS et al (2000) Microsatellite instability in inflammatory bowel disease-associated neoplastic lesions is associated with hypermethylation and diminished expression of the DNA mismatch repair gene, hMLH1. Cancer Res 60(17):4864–4868
139. Hsieh CJ et al (1998) Hypermethylation of the p16INK4a promoter in colectomy specimens of patients with long-standing and extensive ulcerative colitis. Cancer Res 58(17):3942–3945
140. Kominsky DJ et al (2011) An endogenously anti-inflammatory role for methylation in mucosal inflammation identified through metabolite profiling. J Immunol 186 (11):6505–6514
141. O'Hagan HM et al (2011) Oxidative damage targets complexes containing DNA methyltransferases, SIRT1, and polycomb members to promoter CpG Islands. Cancer Cell 20(5):606–619
142. Niwa T et al (2010) Inflammatory processes triggered by Helicobacter pylori infection cause aberrant DNA methylation in gastric epithelial cells. Cancer Res 70(4):1430–1440
143. Katsurano M et al (2012) Early-stage formation of an epigenetic field defect in a mouse colitis model, and non-essential roles of T- and B-cells in DNA methylation induction. Oncogene 31 (3):342–351
144. Lagos-Quintana M et al (2001) Identification of novel genes coding for small expressed RNAs. Science 294(5543):853–858
145. Taft RJ et al (2010) Non-coding RNAs: regulators of disease. J Pathol 220(2):126–139
146. Cortez MA et al (2011) MicroRNAs in body fluids--the mix of hormones and biomarkers. Nat Rev Clin Oncol 8(8):467–477
147. Ludwig K et al (2013) PDCD4/miR-21 dysregulation in inflammatory bowel disease-associated carcinogenesis. Virchows Arch 462(1):57–63
148. Olaru AV et al (2013) MicroRNA-224 negatively regulates p21 expression during late neoplastic progression in inflammatory bowel disease. Inflamm Bowel Dis 19(3):471–480
149. Olaru AV et al (2011) Dynamic changes in the expression of MicroRNA-31 during inflammatory bowel disease-associated neoplastic transformation. Inflamm Bowel Dis 17 (1):221–231
150. Fujii S et al (2005) Methylation of the oestrogen receptor gene in non-neoplastic epithelium as a marker of colorectal neoplasia risk in longstanding and extensive ulcerative colitis. Gut 54(9):1287–1292
151. Tominaga K et al (2005) Prediction of colorectal neoplasia by quantitative methylation analysis of estrogen receptor gene in nonneoplastic epithelium from patients with ulcerative colitis. Clin Cancer Res 11(24 Pt 1):8880–8885
152. Bernstein CN, Shanahan F, Weinstein WM (1994) Are we telling patients the truth about surveillance colonoscopy in ulcerative colitis? Lancet 343(8889):71–74
153. Blackstone MO et al (1981) Dysplasia-associated lesion or mass (DALM) detected by colonoscopy in long-standing ulcerative colitis: an indication for colectomy. Gastroenterology 80(2):366–374
154. Odze RD (1999) Adenomas and adenoma-like DALMs in chronic ulcerative colitis: a clinical, pathological, and molecular review. Am J Gastroenterol 94(7):1746–1750
155. Kiran RP et al (2014) Risk and location of cancer in patients with preoperative colitis-associated dysplasia undergoing proctocolectomy. Ann Surg 259(2):302–309
156. Ullman TA et al (2002) The fate of low grade dysplasia in ulcerative colitis. Am J Gastroenterol 97(4):922–927
157. Sugita A et al (1993) Survival with colorectal cancer in ulcerative colitis. A study of 102 cases. Ann Surg 218(2):189–195
158. Schwarz RJ, Pezim ME (1991) Failure of right-sided coloanal anastomosis for treatment of left-sided ulcerative colitis. Report of a case. Dis Colon Rectum 34(7):618–621
159. Alessandroni L et al (2012) Adenocarcinoma below stapled ileoanal anastomosis after restorative proctocolectomy for ulcerative colitis. Updat Surg 64(2):149–152

160. Sagayama K et al (2007) Incidence of and risk factors for dysplasia in mucosectomy area in ulcerative colitis patients undergoing restorative proctocolectomy. Int J Color Dis 22 (4):439–443
161. Tsunoda A, Talbot IC, Nicholls RJ (1990) Incidence of dysplasia in the anorectal mucosa in patients having restorative proctocolectomy. Br J Surg 77(5):506–508
162. Chia CS et al (2008) Adenocarcinoma of the anal transitional zone after double stapled ileal pouch-anal anastomosis for ulcerative colitis. Color Dis 10(6):621–623
163. Remzi FH et al (2003) Dysplasia of the anal transitional zone after ileal pouch-anal anastomosis: results of prospective evaluation after a minimum of ten years. Dis Colon Rectum 46 (1):6–13
164. Ziv Y et al (1994) Incidence, risk factors, and treatment of dysplasia in the anal transitional zone after ileal pouch-anal anastomosis. Dis Colon Rectum 37(12):1281–1285
165. Galli-Gallardo SM, Pang PK, Oguro C (1979) Renal responses of the chilean toad, Calyptocephalella caudiverbera, and the mud puppy, Necturus maculosus, to mesotocin. Gen Comp Endocrinol 37(1):134–136
166. Remzi FH, Preen M (2003) Rectal cancer and ulcerative colitis: does it change the therapeutic approach? Color Dis 5(5):483–485
167. Pedersen ME et al (2008) Adenocarcinoma arising from the rectal stump eleven years after excision of an ileal J-pouch in a patient with ulcerative colitis: report of a case. Dis Colon Rectum 51(7):1146–1148
168. Radice E et al (1998) Ileal pouch-anal anastomosis in patients with colorectal cancer: long-term functional and oncologic outcomes. Dis Colon Rectum 41(1):11–17
169. Wu XR et al (2013) Preoperative pelvic radiation increases the risk for ileal pouch failure in patients with colitis-associated colorectal cancer. J Crohns Colitis 7(10):e419–e426
170. Selvaggi F et al (2014) Systematic review of cuff and pouch cancer in patients with ileal pelvic pouch for ulcerative colitis. Inflamm Bowel Dis 20(7):1296–1308
171. Derikx LA et al (2014) Prior colorectal neoplasia is associated with increased risk of ileoanal pouch neoplasia in patients with inflammatory bowel disease. Gastroenterology 146 (1):119–128, e1
172. Heuschen UA et al (2001) Adenocarcinoma in the ileal pouch: late risk of cancer after restorative proctocolectomy. Int J Color Dis 16(2):126–130
173. Herfarth C, Heuschen G, Heuschen UA (1998) Malignant transformation in ulcerative colitis and surgical implications. Chirurg 69(10):1020–1027
174. Lofberg R et al (1991) Dysplasia and DNA aneuploidy in a pelvic pouch. Report of a case. Dis Colon Rectum 34(3):280–283, discussion 283–4
175. Veress B et al (1995) Long-term histomorphological surveillance of the pelvic ileal pouch: dysplasia develops in a subgroup of patients. Gastroenterology 109(4):1090–1097
176. Palascak-Juif V et al (2005) Small bowel adenocarcinoma in patients with Crohn's disease compared with small bowel adenocarcinoma de novo. Inflamm Bowel Dis 11(9):828–832
177. Whiteford MH et al (2000) Usefulness of FDG-PET scan in the assessment of suspected metastatic or recurrent adenocarcinoma of the colon and rectum. Dis Colon Rectum 43 (6):759–767, discussion 767–70
178. Connelly TM, Koltun WA (2013) The surgical treatment of inflammatory bowel disease-associated dysplasia. Expert Rev Gastroenterol Hepatol 7(4):307–321, quiz 322
179. Hamilton SR (1985) Colorectal carcinoma in patients with Crohn's disease. Gastroenterology 89(2):398–407
180. Sengul N et al (2006) Effects of radiotherapy on different histopathological types of rectal carcinoma. Color Dis 8(4):283–288
181. Bosset JF et al (2005) Enhanced tumorocidal effect of chemotherapy with preoperative radiotherapy for rectal cancer: preliminary results–EORTC 22921. J Clin Oncol 23 (24):5620–5627
182. Grillo-Ruggieri F et al (2007) Mucinous rectal adenocarcinoma can be associated to tumor downstaging after preoperative chemoradiotherapy. Dis Colon Rectum 50(10):1594–1603

183. Basik M et al (1995) Prognosis and recurrence patterns of anal adenocarcinoma. Am J Surg 169(2):233–237
184. Nelson RL, Prasad ML, Abcarian H (1985) Anal carcinoma presenting as a perirectal abscess or fistula. Arch Surg 120(5):632–635
185. Abel ME et al (1993) Adenocarcinoma of the anal glands. Results of a survey. Dis Colon Rectum 36(4):383–387

Part I
Clinical Features

Chapter 2
Incidence and Risk Factors

Koji Tanaka, Toshimitsu Araki, Yuji Toiyama, Yoshiki Okita, Yasuhiko Mohri, and Masato Kusunoki

Abstract Epidemiological data indicate that inflammatory bowel disease (IBD), including ulcerative colitis (UC) and Crohn's disease (CD), is the third highest risk condition for the development of colorectal cancer (CRC), namely, colitis-associated cancer (CAC). CD is also associated with an increased risk of small-bowel adenocarcinoma, in response to chronic inflammation of the small intestine. In studies published in the 1990s, the risk for CAC in IBD was approximately 7 % at 20 years after diagnosis. In recent studies, the overall incidence of CAC in IBD is lower, less than 5 % at 20 years. However, several factors, such as the longer duration of colitis, extensive or severer colitis, and coexistent primary sclerosing cholangitis, have continued to be important in the development of CRC in patients with IBD. Despite clinical and experimental investigations, the molecular mechanisms by which chronic inflammation promotes cancer progression are still unknown.

Keywords Chronic inflammation • Duration of colitis • Extensive colitis • Primary sclerosing cholangitis

2.1 Inflammatory Bowel Disease

Inflammatory bowel disease (IBD) is an idiopathic inflammatory disorder of the gastrointestinal tract that consists of two major forms: ulcerative colitis (UC) and Crohn's disease (CD) [1]. UC extends proximally from the anal verge and involves the entire colon or a part of it. The inflammation in UC is limited to the mucosal layer. By contrast, CD can affect any part of the gastrointestinal tract but typically involves the distal part of the small intestine (ileum) and the colon. The affected segments frequently show a discontinuous pattern. The inflammation is transmural and extends to all layers of the intestine.

IBD is characterized by episodes of remission and exacerbation. Despite various effective treatments, some patients experience frequent flares of inflammation or

K. Tanaka (✉) • T. Araki • Y. Toiyama • Y. Okita • Y. Mohri • M. Kusunoki
Department of Gastrointestinal and Pediatric Surgery, Mie University Graduate School of Medicine, 2-174 Edobashi, Tsu, Mie 514-8507, Japan
e-mail: qouji@clin.medic.mie-u.ac.jp

M. Kusunoki (ed.), *Colitis-Associated Cancer*, DOI 10.1007/978-4-431-55522-3_2

develop treatment-resistant disease with chronic inflammation. IBD is associated with various intestinal and extraintestinal complications, with one of the most serious being the development of colorectal cancer (CRC) [2]. IBD patients are at a higher risk of CRC than the general population [3], although the pathogenesis of CRC in IBD is unknown.

2.2 Inflammation and Cancer

Chronic inflammation increases the risk of carcinogenesis in various organs [4], and the link between inflammation and cancer development is well recognized. The molecular biology, immune pathobiology, and genetics of IBD-associated CRC are the focuses of intense research [5].

A link between inflammation and cancer was determined approximately 150 years ago, when, in 1863, Rudolf Virchow discovered the presence of leukocytes in neoplastic tissues. He hypothesized that the "lymphoreticular infiltrate" reflected the origin of cancer at sites of chronic inflammation [6].

Epidemiological data also indicate that inflammation plays an important role in the initiation, promotion, and progression of many types of cancer [7]. Distinct host immune cells, cytokines, and chemical mediators participate in all steps of inflammation-related carcinogenesis: tumor initiation, promotion, progression, and metastasis [8]. Among the chronic inflammatory diseases linked to colorectal carcinogenesis, IBD is perhaps the most widely recognized.

2.3 Sporadic and Hereditary Colorectal Cancer

As the third most common malignancy, CRC is a major cause of cancer-related death worldwide [9, 10]. Sporadic CRC, the most common type of CRC, is thought to develop from benign adenomas. Fearon and Vogelstein characterized the development of sporadic CRC in their model of the adenoma→carcinoma sequence, in which genetic abnormalities accumulate in a stepwise manner and ultimately lead to the development of malignancy [11].

Hereditary CRC accounts for 5–10 % of all CRC cases [9, 10] and consists of two major types: familial adenomatous polyposis (FAP) and hereditary nonpolyposis colorectal cancer (HNPCC), also known as Lynch syndrome. FAP is an autosomal-dominant inherited disorder resulting from germ-line mutations in the adenomatous polyposis coli (APC) gene [12]. In patients with FAP, numerous adenomatous polyps develop, mainly in the colon and rectum. Although they are benign, they are at extremely high risk of becoming malignant. HNPCC, or Lynch syndrome, is also an autosomal-dominant inherited syndrome. It results from defective mismatch repair proteins that show high microsatellite instability [13]. Patients with HNPCC have a tendency to develop CRC and are at increased risk of other cancers, such as endometrial, ovarian, gastric, small intestinal, hepatobiliary, pancreatic, upper urinary, prostate, brain, and skin cancers.

2.4 Colitis-Associated Cancer

IBD-associated CRC, or colitis-associated cancer (CAC), is a form of CRC arising in patients with IBD [14]. Chronic inflammation of the large bowel such as that which occurs in IBD is associated with the subsequent development of CRC [15], as the repeated flare-ups of inflammation characteristic of IBD often lead to oncogenic insults to colonic epithelial cells.

In 1925, Crohn and Rosenberg reported a case of rectal carcinoma complicating UC and postulated that the lesion developed as a late manifestation of UC [16]. In 1948, Warren and Sommers reported a case of adenocarcinoma of the ascending colon in a patient with CD complicating regional enteritis [17]. Much later, in 2005, CD was also shown to be associated with an increased risk of small-bowel adenocarcinoma, due to chronic inflammation of the small intestine [18].

IBD is the third highest risk condition for the development of CRC, after FAP and HNPCC. Unlike sporadic and hereditary CRC, CAC usually derives from a focal or multifocal dysplastic mucosa in areas of chronic inflammation via an inflammation→dysplasia→carcinoma sequence [2]. CAC accounts for 1–2 % of all cases of CRC and for 10–15 % of all deaths among IBD patients. It is thus one of the most important causes of mortality in IBD patients [1, 2].

2.5 Clinical Features of CAC

The clinical features of CAC are distinct from those of sporadic CRC and are reviewed below.

2.5.1 Age at Diagnosis

The mean age of CAC development in IBD patients is lower than that of sporadic CRC in the general population.

Several studies have examined the age of CAC development in patients with UC. In the meta-analysis by Eaden et al. [19], the mean age at UC-CAC diagnosis was 43.2 years. Lakatos et al. [20] reported a median age of 51 years at the time of UC-CAC diagnosis, which, in Hungary, is almost 15 years younger than that of sporadic CRC development in the general population. In the study of Watanabe et al. [21], the mean age at UC-CAC diagnosis was 56.8 years, younger than the

62.5 years of patients in the Japanese general population who are newly diagnosed with sporadic CRC.

2.6 Pathological Features of CAC

CAC frequently progresses from flat or nonpolypoid dysplasia to invasive adenocarcinoma. The tumors show aggressive growth and early metastasis [22].

In patients with UC, the rectum and the sigmoid colon are the most common sites of CAC. Compared with the general population, CAC arising in UC patients shows a more proximal distribution in the colon. Watanabe et al. [21] showed that UC-CAC tended to be of a higher histologic grade, such as mucinous or signet ring cell type, and had a greater frequency of developing as multiple synchronous CRCs.

In CD patients, CAC is evenly distributed between the different colonic segments [22].

2.7 Prognosis of CAC

The prognosis for patients with sporadic CRC and CAC is very similar, with 5-year survival rates of 50–60 % [21, 22].

In the study of Watanabe et al. [21], the 5-year overall survival rates of patients with UC-CAC and sporadic CRC were 64.2 % and 68.7 % ($P = 0.585$), respectively. According to Delaunoit et al. [23], 5-year survival rates were 54 % in patients with UC-CAC and 53 % in those with sporadic CRC ($P = 0.94$). However, patients with stage III UC-CAC were shown to have a significantly lower 5-year overall survival rate than those with sporadic CRC (43.3 % vs 57.4 %, $P = 0.032$), whereas the differences for stages I, II, and IV were not significant. Watanabe et al. [21] similarly concluded that the prognosis of patients with advanced-stage UC-CAC is poorer than that of patients with sporadic CRC.

2.8 Molecular Mechanisms of CAC Development

The premalignant lesion→carcinoma sequence of both sporadic CRC and CAC suggests the involvement of multiple gene alterations as the mechanism leading to carcinogenesis [24]. However, CAC differs from sporadic CRC with respect to tumor biology and the pathways leading to malignancy.

Sporadic CRC develops from a premalignant adenoma(s) through mutations in genes such as APC, KRAS (Kirsten rat sarcoma viral oncogene homolog), p53, and DCC (deleted in colorectal carcinoma netrin 1 receptor) [25]. In CAC, tumorigenesis is via a transition from low- to high-grade dysplasia, although multiple gene alterations are likewise involved [26]. However, there are significant differences in the timing and frequency of the gene alterations leading to sporadic CRC vs CAC.

2.8.1 *APC*

In sporadic CRC, mutations in the tumor suppressor gene APC have been identified as one of the earliest genetic alterations in the pathogenesis of CRC. APC gene mutations are also found in CAC but generally as much later genetic events.

In the series of Aust et al. [27], one (3 %) out of 30 UC-CAC patients had an APC mutation compared with 11 (26 %) of the 42 patients with sporadic CRC. Similarly, in the study of Tarmin et al. [28], two (6 %) of their 33 patients with UC-associated dysplasia and CAC had a total of three truncating APC mutations compared with 17 (74 %) of the 23 patients with sporadic CRC. The results of these two studies suggest that the loss of APC function is a common initiating event in sporadic CRC but not in CAC.

2.8.2 *p53*

In sporadic CRC, p53 late-developing mutations are characteristic of morphologically aggressive lesions. Loss of p53 function occurs in approximately 85 % of CAC and is an important step in CAC progression. Mutations in p53 are found not only in dysplastic or malignant cells but also in chronically inflamed nondysplastic mucosa, suggesting that they are an early genetic event in the pathogenesis of CAC [29].

2.8.3 *KRAS*

KRAS mutations are another early genetic event in the pathogenesis of CAC [30].

2.9 Incidence of CRC in IBD

Table 2.1 summarizes the incidence of CAC in patients with IBD, and Table 2.2 the incidence of CAC and small-bowel cancer in those with CD.

In studies published in the 1980s to 1990s, the risk for CRC in UC was around 7 % 20 years after UC diagnosis [31] and around 14 % at 25 years [32, 33]. In the

Table 2.1 Incidence of colitis-associated cancer in inflammatory bowel disease (IBD)

Author	Year of publication	Type of study	IBD patients	No. of CAC patients	Incidence or risk ratios
Eaden et al. [19]	2001	Meta-analysis	UC	1,698	10 years, 1.6; 20 years, 8.3; 30 years, 18.4 %
Jess et al. [36]	2012	Meta-analysis	UC	229	10 years, <1 %; 15 years, 0.2–2.0 %; 20 years, 1.1–5.3 %
Lutgens et al. [37]	2013	Meta-analysis	UC and CD	NA	10 years, 1 %; 20 years, 2 %; >20 years, 5 %
Ekbom et al. [45]	1990	Population based	UC	91	5.7 (1958–1984)
Winther et al. [34]	2004	Population-based cohort	UC	124	10 years, 0.4 %; 20 years, 1.1 %; 30 years, 2.1 %
Rutter et al. [35]	2006	Prospective	UC	30	20 years, 2.5 %; 30 years, 7.6 %; 40 years, 10.8 %
Lakatos et al. [20]	2006	Population based	UC	13	10 years, 0.6 %; 20 years, 5.4 %; 30 years, 7.5 %
Söderlund et al. [41]	2009	Population based	UC and CD	188	10 years, 1 %; 20 years, 1.5 %; 30 years, 2.7 %
Jess et al. [42]	2012	Nationwide survey	UC and CD	UC: 268, CD: 70	1.34 (1979–1988), 0.57 (1999–2008)
Manninen et al. [43]	2013	Population based	UC and CD	21	1.83 in IBD, 1.99 in UC, 1.82 in CD

CAC, colitis-associated cancer; UC, ulcerative colitis; CD, Crohn's disease; NA, not available

Table 2.2 Incidence of colitis-associated cancer in Crohn's disease (CD)

Author	Year of publication	Type of study	IBD patients	Risk of CAC	Risk of small-bowel cancer
Jess et al. [18]	2005	Meta-analysis	CD	0.9–2.2	3.4–66.7
Canavan et al. [38]	2006	Meta-analysis	CD	2.5	33.2
von Roon et al. [39]	2007	Meta-analysis	CD	2.4	28.4
Laukoetter et al. [40]	2011	Meta-analysis	CD	0.5 person-years	0.3 person-years
Lovasz et al. [44]	2013	Population-based cohort	CD	7.73	NA

IBD, inflammatory bowel disease; NA, not available

early 2000s, the probability of developing CRC in UC was 1.6 % at 10 years, 8.3 % at 20 years, and 18.4 % at 30 years [19]. According to more recent data, the cumulative incidences of CRC in UC are approximately 1.0 % at 10 years, 2.0–5.0 % at 20 years, and 5.0–7.5 % at 30 years [20, 34, 35]. The decreased incidence of CAC in IBD may be because of the improved therapeutic management of colitis, with higher rates of mucosal healing, but definitive clinical and experimental evidence supporting these observations is lacking.

Because chronic inflammation of the large bowel is an important factor in the development of CRC, anti-inflammatory agents have been considered as chemopreventive agents.

2.9.1 Meta-analysis of the Incidence of CRC in UC

The reported incidence varies widely between studies, which reflects the different periods of data collection, different methodologies, and data originating from studies in different countries. The results of the three meta-analyses published in the English-language literature are summarized briefly below.

Eaden et al. [19] accumulated the results of 116 studies comprising 54,478 patients with UC. In this cohort, there were 1,698 cases of CRC. The probability of developing CRC 10 years after UC diagnosis was 1.6 %, rising to 8.3 % after 20 years and 18.4 % after 30 years. The overall prevalence of CAC in UC in that series was 3.7 %, increasing to 5.4 % in patients with pancolitis. The data pointed to an association between the extent of colitis and the increased risk of CAC.

Jess et al. [36] carried out a meta-analysis of eight studies on the basis of strict inclusion and exclusion criteria. During 14 years of follow-up, 1.6 % of the patients in their study were diagnosed with UC-CAC. The pooled standardized incidence ratio (SIR) was 2.4 (range, 1.05–3.1). The cumulative incidences of CRC development were <1.0 % at 10 years, 0.4–2 % at 15 years, and 1.1–5.3 % at 20 years of follow-up. The sex-specific risk ratio was 1.9 in females and 2.6 in males. The age-specific risk ratio was 8.6 in patients 0–39 years of age, 2.1 in those 40–60 years of age, and 1.7 in those 60 years of age and older. Patients with extensive colitis and pancolitis (beyond proctosigmoiditis) had a 4.8-fold higher risk of UC-CAC.

Lutgens et al. [37] reported that the pooled SIR of CRC in IBD patients was 1.7 (range, 1.2–2.2). The cumulative risk of CRC was 1 %, 2 %, and 5 % after 10, 20, and >20 years of disease duration, respectively. The authors concluded that the risk of CRC in IBD patients is significantly higher in patients with longer disease duration, extensive disease, and IBD diagnosed at a young age.

2.9.2 Meta-analysis of the Incidence of CRC in CD

In an earlier meta-analysis, Jess et al. [18] evaluated six population-based studies in which the incidence of intestinal malignancies in CD patients was examined. The overall pooled risk estimates (SIRs) for CRCs in CD ranged from 0.9 to 2.2. The SIR for small-bowel cancer ranged from 3.4 to 66.7. The overall pooled estimate for intestinal malignancies in CD was 27.1. These results showed that CD patients have an overall higher risk of CRC and small-bowel cancer.

Canavan et al. [38] accumulated the results of 13 studies comprising 11,840 patients with CD to examine the incidence of intestinal malignancies in that group. The overall relative risk (RR) of CRC in CD was 2.5 (range, 1.3–4.7). The risk of CRC in CD was shown to be significantly higher than in the general population but not significantly different from that in UC. The cumulative RR for CRC development in CD was 2.9 % at 10 years after CD diagnosis, 5.6 % at 20 years, and 8.3 % at 30 years. However, the authors also found that the overall RR for small-bowel cancer in CD was 33.2 (range, 15.9–60.9). Thus, the risk of small-bowel cancer is much higher in CD patients than in the general population.

Von Roon et al. [39] accumulated the results of 34 studies with a total of 60,122 patients with CD. Compared with the baseline general population, the RRs of CRC and small-bowel cancer were 2.4 (95 % confidence interval, 1.6–4.4) and 28.4 (95 % confidence interval, 14.5–55.7), respectively.

Laukoetter et al. [40] analyzed the results of 20 studies comprising 40,547 patients with CD. The incidence of CD-associated cancer (CDAC) was 0.8/1,000 person-years, meaning that during a 1-year observation period, 0.8 CD patients out of 1,000 developed CDAC. The incidence of CRC and small-bowel carcinoma in CD was 0.5/1,000 and 0.5/1,000 person-years, respectively. The mean age at CRC diagnosis in CD patients was 51.5 years, which is 20 years earlier than in the general population. The mean duration between CD diagnosis and CDAC was 18.3 years.

2.9.3 Incidence of CRC in IBD in a Population-Based Cohort Study

S-derlund et al. [41] assessed cancer occurrence and cancer-related mortality in 7,607 Swedish IBD patients in a population-based cohort study. CRC was detected in 188 IBD patients during 198,227 person-years of follow-up. Compared with the general population, the incidence of CRC in IBD corresponded to an overall twofold higher risk (SIR, 2.3). The overall cumulative incidence of CRC in IBD at 10, 20, and 30 years after IBD diagnosis was 1 %, 1.5 %, and 2.7 %, respectively.

Jess et al. [42] studied CRC risk in a nationwide cohort of 47,374 Danish patients with IBD over a 30-year period. Over the course of the follow-up evaluation, 268 patients with UC (0.5 %) and 70 patients with CD (0.1 %) developed CRC. The overall RR of CRC in UC patients was comparable to that of the general population (RR = 1.1), whereas the RR of CRC in CD patients was slightly lower (0.9) but did not change significantly over time. In UC patients, the overall RR for CRCs decreased from 1.34 between 1979 and 1988 to 0.57 between 1999 and 2008.

Manninen et al. [43] studied the risk of CRC in a nationwide cohort of 1,915 Finnish patients with IBD (1,254 with UC, 550 with CD, and 111 with inflammatory bowel unclassified). CRC was found in 21 patients. The SIR was 1.83 for IBD, 1.99 for UC, and 1.92 for CD.

Lovasz et al. [44] examined the CRC risk in 640 CD patients with colonic involvement and stenosing disease in a population-based cohort from Hungary. CRC was diagnosed in six CD patients during a follow-up of 7,759 person-years. The mean overall CRC incidence rate was 7.73 per 10,000 patient-years.

2.9.4 Incidence of CRC in UC in a Population-Based Cohort Study

Ekbom et al. [45] examined a population-based cohort of 3,117 patients with UC. In 91 patients with UC, there were 92 cases of CRC (2.9 %). Compared with the general population, the RR for CRC was 1.7 for patients with proctitis, 2.8 for those with left-sided colitis, and 14.8 for those with pancolitis. Less extensive colitis at diagnosis was associated with a lower risk of CRC development.

Winther et al. [34] evaluated a population-based cohort of 1,160 patients with UC in Copenhagen County. After a follow-up of up to 36 years, there were 124 malignancies (10.7 %). The cumulative probability of CRC was 0.4 % by 10 years, 1.1 % by 20 years, and 2.1 % by 30 years of disease. The authors concluded that neither the overall cancer risk nor the risk of CAC was increased after a median of 19 years of follow-up. In their analysis of surgical intervention, the overall cumulative probability of colectomy was 21.3 % after 10 years, 27.9 % after 20 years, 29.9 % after 30 years, and 31.[illegible] % after 35 years. This is in contrast to a rate of 9.1–16.4 % in the cohort reported by Eaden et al. [19]. An active surgical approach after medical treatment failure may explain the low rate of CRC development in the former study.

Rutter et al. [35] examined 600 patients who underwent 2,627 colonoscopic surveillance procedures over a 30-year period, during which 74 patients (12.3 %) developed neoplasia, including 30 cases of CRC (5 %). The cumulative incidence of CRC by colitis duration was 2.5 % at 20 years, 7.6 % at 30 years, and 10.8 % at 40 years. During the surveillance program, 89 patients (14.8 % of the study population) underwent colonic surgery.

Lakatos et al. [20] evaluated the relevant epidemiological and clinical data of 723 UC patients in a Hungarian population-based cohort study. CRC was detected in 13 patients (8,564-person-year duration). The cumulative risk of developing CRC after a 10-year duration of colitis was 0.6 %, which increased to 5.4 % at 20 years and 7.5 % at 30 years.

2.10 Risk Factors for CAC

The increased risk of CAC in IBD patients is thought to be due to genetic and acquired factors (Table 2.3), including the duration, extent, and severity of colitis, the presence of post-inflammatory polyps (pseudopolyps), young age at onset of colitis, sex, family history of sporadic CRC, coexistence of primary sclerosing cholangitis and/or colonic strictures, and the presence of colonic dysplasia. Of these, the most important and well-recognized risk factors for CAC are the duration and extent of colitis.

2.10.1 Duration of Colitis

The importance of colitis duration as a risk factor for the development of CRC in IBD patients is supported by several studies, including the above-cited studies of Eaden et al. [19] (Sect. 2.9.1), Lakatos et al. [20] (Sect. 2.9.4), and Rutter et al. [35] (Sect. 2.9.4). In the study of Lakatos et al. [20], a longer duration of colitis (10 years) was identified as a risk factor for developing CRC, according to a logistic regression model (odds ratio, 8.3; $P = 0.04$). Nieminen et al. [46] examined 183 IBD patients with dysplasia or CRC and 368 matched control patients in a case-control study. They concluded that an increasing degree of inflammation and disease duration cumulatively increased the risk of dysplasia in IBD.

Table 2.3 Risk factors for colitis-associated cancer

Risk factor	Relevant references
Duration of colitis	Eaden et al. [19]; Lakatos et al. [20]; Rutter et al. [35]; Nieminen et al. [46]
Extent of colitis	Ekbom et al. [45]; Eaden et al. [19]; Lakatos et al. [20]; Söderlund et al. [41]; Jess et al. [36]
Severity of colitis	Rutter et al. [47]; Gupta et al. [48]
Post-inflammatory polyps	Rutter et al. [47]; Velayos et al. [49]; Baars et al. [50]
Young age at onset of colitis	Ekbom et al. [45]; Eaden et al. [19]; Jess et al. [36]
Sex	Jess et al. [42]; Ekbom et al. [45]
Family history of sporadic colorectal cancer	Askling et al. [51]; Velayos et al. [49]
Primary sclerosing cholangitis	Broomé et al. [56]; Soetikno et al. [57] Lakatos et al. [20]; Loftus et al. [58]; Nuako et al. [59]
Colonic stricture	Rutter et al. [47]
Colonic dysplasia	Lakatos et al. [20]

2.10.2 Extent of Colitis

Current evidence suggests that the risk of CAC begins to increase after 8–10 years of extensive colitis, defined as left-sided colitis extending from the anal verge to the splenic flexure, and pancolitis (beyond the splenic flexure). By contrast, several studies have shown that there is little or no increased risk of CRC in patients with proctitis or proctosigmoiditis. Chronic colonic inflammation presumably leads to dysplasia and thus eventually to cancer.

The relationship between the extent of colitis and CRC was cited in the abovementioned study of Ekbom et al. [45] (Sect. 2.9.4). In the study of Eaden et al. [19], among UC patients with pancolitis, the cumulative incidence of CRC was 2.1 % at 10 years, 8.5 % at 20 years, and 17.8 % at 30 years disease duration. These data are very similar to the cumulative incidence of CRC in all UC patients, indicating that the development of CRC in UC is associated with pancolitis.

In their univariate analysis, Lakatos et al. [20] showed that patients with pancolitis had a higher risk of CRC than those with left-sided colitis (odds ratio, 5.3; $P = 0.001$). Pancolitis was also identified as a risk factor for CRC development in their logistic regression model (odds ratio, 1.8; $P = 0.04$).

In the above-cited study of Söderlund et al. [41] (Sect. 2.9.3), compared with the general population, the RR of CRC was 2.7 for all UC patients and 5.6 for those with pancolitis. Compared with patients with UC proctitis (RR = 1), the RR of incident CRC was 1.2 for patients with left-sided colitis and 2.0 for those with pancolitis. These data suggest that the greater the extent of colitis, the greater the risk of CRC.

In their meta-analysis (see Sect. 2.9.1), Jess et al. [36] demonstrated that patients with extensive colitis and pancolitis had a 4.8 times higher risk of UC-CAC.

2.10.3 Severity of Colitis

Several reports have demonstrated a significant correlation between the severity of colitis and the risk of CAC, in which chronic inflammation is believed to initiate and promote carcinogenesis in various organs.

Rutter et al. [47] studied 68 patients with CRC and 136 control patients who were matched with respect to sex, extent of colitis, age at diagnosis, duration of colitis, and year of index surveillance colonoscopy. In a multivariate analysis, the authors demonstrated that the histologic severity of colitis was an independent risk factor for the development of CRC (odds ratio, 4.7; $P < 0.001$). A multivariate analysis also showed that a macroscopically normal colonoscopy examination was an independent factor for a lower risk of CRC development (odds ratio, 0.38; $P = 0.003$).

Gupta et al. [48] examined 418 patients with no initial dysplasia who underwent regular endoscopic surveillance. Among them, 15 (3.6 %) progressed to advanced neoplasia (high-grade dysplasia or colorectal cancer). The authors found a significant relationship between histologic inflammation over time and progression to advanced neoplasia. According to a multivariate analysis, the microscopically determined severity of inflammation was an independent risk factor for developing advanced colorectal neoplasia.

2.10.4 Post-inflammatory Polyps (Pseudopolyps)

Post-inflammatory polyps (colonic pseudopolyps) are irregular islands of colonic mucosa that form by colonic inflammation and regeneration. They are not premalignant lesions and in themselves have no malignant potential. Rather, the presence of post-inflammatory polyps is thought to be a historical marker of previous severe inflammation. As such, they are a known risk factor for CAC.

In the above-cited study of Rutter et al. [47] (Sect. 2.10.3), patients with post-inflammatory polyps had a higher risk of CRC, according to both a univariate (odds ratio, 2.1; $P = 0.006$) and a multivariate (odds ratio, 2.3; $P = 0.005$) analysis.

In a case-control study, Velayos et al. [49] evaluated 188 UC patients with CRC and 188 matched control patients. Based on a univariate analysis, there was a significant association between a prior diagnosis of pseudopolyps and CRC (odds ratio, 2.0; $P < 0.05$), even after adjusting for surveillance colonoscopy and anti-inflammatory therapy (odds ratio, 2.5; $P < 0.05$). These results suggested that a history of post-inflammatory pseudopolyps is a predictive factor for CRC in UC patients.

However, Baars et al. [50] studied the characteristics of IBD-related CRC in a nationwide IBD cohort, in which 251cases of IBD-related CRC were diagnosed (UC, $n = 171$; CD, $n = 77$; unclassified colitis, $n = 3$). The median time from IBD diagnosis to CRC diagnosis was 12 years. Type of IBD, sex of the patient, concomitant PSC, pseudopolyps, extent of inflammation, and medication use were not related to early CRCs that developed within 8 years after the diagnosis of IBD.

2.10.5 Young Age at Onset of Colitis

Young age at colitis onset is recognized as a risk factor for the development of CAC. Ekbom et al. [45] found that the RR of CRC decreased for each increase in age at diagnosis (under 15 years, 15–29 years, 30–39 years, 40–49 years, 50–59 years, and ≥60 years). For patients with extensive disease after 35 years of colitis, the cumulative risk for CRC was 40 % for those diagnosed under the age of 15 years and 25 % for those diagnosed at 15–39 years of age.

Eaden et al. [19] analyzed the incidence of CRC in children diagnosed with UC (average age at UC onset, 10 years). Within this group, the cumulative risk of CRC was 5.5 % at 10 years, 10.8 % at 20 years, and 15.7 % at 30 years. These rates are higher than the corresponding rates for adults (3 %, 5.9 %, and 8.7 %, respectively).

In the above-cited meta-analysis of Jess et al. [36] (Sect. 2.9.1), the age-specific risk ratio was 8.6, 2.1, and 1.7 in patients 0–39, 40–60, and ≥60 years of age, respectively. Thus, young age at UC diagnosis increased the risk of CRC in UC patients.

2.10.6 *Sex*

The association between sex and the risk of CRC in IBD has been reported. Jess et al. [36] reported a sex-specific risk ratio of 1.9 in females and 2.6 in males. Ekbom et al. [45] showed a similar risk for IBD-CRC in males and females. Among patients with UC, the RR was 5.6 and 5.9, respectively. In those with CD, the RR was 2.8 and 2.1, respectively.

2.10.7 *Family History of Sporadic CRC*

Askling et al. [51] assessed the significance of a family history of CRC on the risk of CRC in a population-based cohort study of 19,876 patients with UC or CD. A family history of CRC was associated with a more than twofold risk of CRC (adjusted RR = 2.5). Patients with a first-degree relative diagnosed with CRC before age 50 years also had a higher risk (RR = 9.2).

In the abovementioned case-control study of Velayos et al. [49] (Sect. 2.10.4), a family history of CRC was an independent risk factor for IBD-CRC in patients with UC (odds ratio, 3.7).

2.10.8 *Coexistent Primary Sclerosing Cholangitis*

Primary sclerosing cholangitis (PSC) is a chronic cholestatic hepatobiliary disease characterized by inflammation and fibrosis of the intrahepatic and extrahepatic biliary tract [52]. PSC causes multiple intrahepatic and extrahepatic biliary strictures, resulting in cholestasis, liver cirrhosis, portal hypertension, and liver failure. Its etiology is thus far unknown, but autoimmunity is thought to be the main cause.

The incidence of IBD in patients with PSC is 25–30 %. However, the association between PSC and CD is relatively rare, such that 85–90 % of the patients with PSC and IBD are those with UC [53].

The association between PSC and CD was first reported by Atkinson and Carroll [54], in 1964, and between PSC and UC by Smith and Loe [55], in 1965. Since then, many studies have identified PSC as a risk factor for the development of CRC in patients with UC. In the study by Broomé et al. [56], five (28 %) of the 17 UC patients who developed dysplasia or carcinoma had PSC. Soetikno et al. [57] performed a meta-analysis of 11 studies comprising 16,844 patients with UC. Overall, 21 % of the patients with both UC and PSC developed colorectal neoplasms, compared with 4 % of the UC patients without PSC. Among patients with PSC, the RR of developing dysplasia or cancer was 4.8. In both a univariate analysis and a logistic regression model, Lakatos et al. [20] showed that patients with PSC had a higher risk of CRCs (odds ratio, 27.1 and 9.5, respectively). However, these results of an association between PSC and an increased risk of CRC in UC have been contradicted by others [58,59].

2.10.9 Colonic Strictures

In their case-control study of 68 patients with UC and colorectal neoplasia and 136 matched control patients, Rutter et al. [47] found that colonic strictures increased the risk of colorectal neoplasia in UC (odds ratio, 4.62).

2.10.10 Colonic Dysplasia

As noted above, the premalignant histological changes in UC develop from dysplasia rather than adenoma. Adenocarcinoma of the colon develops from a dysplastic precursor lesion. In their univariate analysis and in a logistic regression model, Lakatos et al. [20] showed that patients with dysplasia had a higher risk of CRC (odds ratio, 19.3; $P = 0.0001$ and odds ratio 4.72; $P = 0.05$, respectively).

References

1. Mattar MC, Lough D, Pishvaian MJ et al (2011) Current management of inflammatory bowel disease and colorectal cancer. Gastrointest Cancer Res 4:53–61
2. Rubin DC, Shaker A, Levin MS (2012) Chronic intestinal inflammation: inflammatory bowel disease and colitis-associated colon cancer. Front Immunol 20123:107
3. Rogler G (2014) Chronic ulcerative colitis and colorectal cancer. Cancer Lett 345:235–241
4. Colotta F, Allavena P, Sica A et al (2009) Cancer-related inflammation, the seventh hallmark of cancer: links to genetic instability. Carcinogenesis 30:1073–1081
5. Atsumi T, Singh R, Sabharwal L et al (2014) Inflammation amplifier, a new paradigm in cancer biology. Cancer Res 74:8–14
6. Balkwill F, Mantovani A (2001) Inflammation and cancer: back to Virchow? Lancet 357:539–545
7. Multhoff G, Molls M, Radons J (2012) Chronic inflammation in cancer development. Front Immunol 2:98

8. Grivennikov SI, Greten FR, Karin M (2010) Immunity, inflammation, and cancer. Cell 140:883–899
9. Brenner H, Kloor M, Pox CP (2014) Colorectal cancer. Lancet 383:1490–1502
10. Markowitz SD, Bertagnolli MM (2009) Molecular origins of cancer: Molecular basis of colorectal cancer. N Engl J Med 361:2449–2460
11. Fearon ER, Vogelstein B (1990) A genetic model for colorectal tumorigenesis. Cell 61:759–767
12. Barrow P, Khan M, Lalloo F et al (2013) Systematic review of the impact of registration and screening on colorectal cancer incidence and mortality in familial adenomatous polyposis and Lynch syndrome. Br J Surg 100:1719–1731
13. Giardiello FM, Allen JI, Axilbund JE et al (2014) Guidelines on genetic evaluation and management of Lynch syndrome: a consensus statement by the US Multi-Society Task Force on colorectal cancer. Gastroenterology 147:502–526
14. Kulaylat MN, Dayton MT (2010) Ulcerative colitis and cancer. J Surg Oncol 101:706–712
15. Kim ER, Chang DK (2014) Colorectal cancer in inflammatory bowel disease: The risk, pathogenesis, prevention and diagnosis. World J Gastroenterol 20:9872–9881
16. Crohn B, Rosenberg H (1925) The sigmoidoscopic picture of chronic ulcerative colitis (non-specific). Am J Med Sci 170:220–228
17. Warren S, Sommers SC (1948) Cicatrizing enteritis (regional ileitis) as a pathologic entity. Am J Pathol 24:475–501
18. Jess T, Gamborg M, Matzen P et al (2005) Increased risk of intestinal cancer in Crohn's disease: a meta-analysis of population-based cohort studies. Am J Gastroenterol 100:2724–2729
19. Eaden JA, Abrams KR, Mayberry JF (2001) The risk of colorectal cancer in ulcerative colitis: a meta-analysis. Gut 48:526–535
20. Lakatos L, Mester G, Erdelyi Z et al (2006) Risk factors for ulcerative colitis-associated colorectal cancer in a Hungarian cohort of patients with ulcerative colitis: results of a population-based study. Inflamm Bowel Dis 12:205–211
21. Watanabe T, Konishi T, Kishimoto J et al (2011) Ulcerative colitis-associated colorectal cancer shows a poorer survival than sporadic colorectal cancer: a nationwide Japanese study. Inflamm Bowel Dis 2011(17):802–808
22. Ren LL, Fang JY (2011) Should we sound the alarm? Dysplasia and colitis-associated colorectal cancer. Asian Pac J Cancer Prev 12:1881–1886
23. Delaunoit T, Limburg PJ, Goldberg RM et al (2006) Colorectal cancer prognosis among patients with inflammatory bowel disease. Clin Gastroenterol Hepatol 4:335–342
24. Kaemmerer E, Klaus C, Jeon MK et al (2013) Molecular classification of colorectal carcinomas: the genotype-to-phenotype relation. World J Gastroenterol 19:8163–8167
25. Fearon ER (2011) Molecular genetics of colorectal cancer. Annu Rev Pathol 6:479–507
26. Hartnett L, Egan LJ (2012) Inflammation, DNA methylation and colitis-associated cancer. Carcinogenesis 33:723–731
27. Aust DE, Terdiman JP, Willenbucher RF et al (2002) The APC/beta-catenin pathway in ulcerative colitis-related colorectal carcinomas: a mutational analysis. Cancer 94:1421–1427
28. Tarmin L, Yin J, Harpaz N et al (1995) Adenomatous polyposis coli gene mutations in ulcerative colitis-associated dysplasias and cancers versus sporadic colon neoplasms. Cancer Res 55:2035–2038
29. Hussain SP, Amstad P, Raja K et al (2000) Increased p53 mutation load in noncancerous colon tissue from ulcerative colitis: a cancer-prone chronic inflammatory disease. Cancer Res 60:3333–3337
30. Benhattar J, Saraga E (1995) Molecular genetics of dysplasia in ulcerative colitis. Eur J Cancer 31A:1171–1173
31. Gyde SN, Prior P, Allan RN et al (1988) Colorectal cancer in ulcerative colitis: a cohort study of primary referrals from three centres. Gut 29:206–217

32. Löfberg R, Broström O, Karlén P et al (1990) Colonoscopic surveillance in long-standing total ulcerative colitis--a 15-year follow-up study. Gastroenterology 99:1021–1031
33. Collins RH Jr, Feldman M, Fordtran JS (1987) Colon cancer, dysplasia, and surveillance in patients with ulcerative colitis. A critical review. N Engl J Med 316:1654–1658
34. Winther KV, Jess T, Langholz E et al (2004) Long-term risk of cancer in ulcerative colitis: a population-based cohort study from Copenhagen County. Clin Gastroenterol Hepatol 2:1088–1095
35. Rutter MD, Saunders BP, Wilkinson KH et al (2006) Thirty-year analysis of a colonoscopic surveillance program for neoplasia in ulcerative colitis. Gastroenterology 130:1030–1038
36. Jess T, Rungoe C, Peyrin-Biroulet L (2012) Risk of colorectal cancer in patients with ulcerative colitis: a meta-analysis of population-based cohort studies. Clin Gastroenterol Hepatol 10:639–645
37. Lutgens MW, van Oijen MG, van der Heijden GJ et al (2013) Declining risk of colorectal cancer in inflammatory bowel disease: an updated meta-analysis of population-based cohort studies. Inflamm Bowel Dis 19:789–799
38. Canavan C, Abrams KR, Mayberry J (2006) Meta-analysis: colorectal and small bowel cancer risk in patients with Crohn's disease. Aliment Pharmacol Ther 23:1097–1104
39. von Roon AC, Reese G, Teare J et al (2007) The risk of cancer in patients with Crohn's disease. Dis Colon Rectum 50:839–855
40. Laukoetter MG, Mennigen R, Hannig CM et al (2011) Intestinal cancer risk in Crohn's disease: a meta-analysis. J Gastrointest Surg 15:576–583
41. Söderlund S, Brandt L, Lapidus A et al (2009) Decreasing time-trends of colorectal cancer in a large cohort of patients with inflammatory bowel disease. Gastroenterology 136:1561–1567
42. Jess T, Simonsen J, Jørgensen KT et al (2012) Decreasing risk of colorectal cancer in patients with inflammatory bowel disease over 30 years. Gastroenterology 143:375–381
43. Manninen P, Karvonen AL, Huhtala H et al (2013) The risk of colorectal cancer in patients with inflammatory bowel diseases in Finland: a follow-up of 20 years. J Crohns Colitis 7:e551–e557
44. Lovasz BD, Lakatos L, Golovics PA et al (2013) Risk of colorectal cancer in Crohn's disease patients with colonic involvement and stenosing disease in a population-based cohort from Hungary. J Gastrointestin Liver Dis 22:265–268
45. Ekbom A, Helmick C, Zack M et al (1990) Ulcerative colitis and colorectal cancer. A population-based study. N Engl J Med 323:1228–1233
46. Nieminen U, Jussila A, Nordling S et al (2014) Inflammation and disease duration have a cumulative effect on the risk of dysplasia and carcinoma in IBD: a case-control observational study based on registry data. Int J Cancer 134:189–196
47. Rutter MD, Saunders BP, Wilkinson KH et al (2004) Cancer surveillance in longstanding ulcerative colitis: endoscopic appearances help predict cancer risk. Gut 53:1813–1816
48. Gupta RB, Harpaz N, Itzkowitz S et al (2007) Histologic inflammation is a risk factor for progression to colorectal neoplasia in ulcerative colitis: a cohort study. Gastroenterology 133:1099–1105
49. Velayos FS, Loftus EV Jr, Jess T et al (2006) Predictive and protective factors associated with colorectal cancer in ulcerative colitis: A case-control study. Gastroenterology 130:1941–1949
50. Baars JE, Kuipers EJ, van Haastert M et al (2012) Age at diagnosis of inflammatory bowel disease influences early development of colorectal cancer in inflammatory bowel disease patients: a nationwide, long-term survey. J Gastroenterol 47:1308–1322
51. Askling J, Dickman PW, Karlén P et al (2001) Family history as a risk factor for colorectal cancer in inflammatory bowel disease. Gastroenterology 120:1356–1362
52. Wang R, Leong RW (2014) Primary sclerosing cholangitis as an independent risk factor for colorectal cancer in the context of inflammatory bowel disease: a review of the literature. World J Gastroenterol 20:8783–8789
53. Tsaitas C, Semertzidou A, Sinakos E (2014) Update on inflammatory bowel disease in patients with primary sclerosing cholangitis. World J Hepatol 6:178–187

54. Atkinson AJ, Carroll WW (1964) Sclerosing cholangitis. Association with regional enteritis. JAMA 188:183–184
55. Smith MP, Loe RJ (1965) Sclerosing cholangitis; review of recent case reports and associated diseases and four new cases. Am J Surg 110:239–246
56. Broomé U, Lindberg G, Löfberg R (1992) Primary sclerosing cholangitis in ulcerative colitis--a risk factor for the development of dysplasia and DNA aneuploidy? Gastroenterology 102:1877–1880
57. Soetikno RM, Lin OS, Heidenreich PA et al (2002) Increased risk of colorectal neoplasia in patients with primary sclerosing cholangitis and ulcerative colitis: a meta-analysis. Gastrointest Endosc 56:48–54
58. Loftus EV Jr, Sandborn WJ, Tremaine WJ et al (1996) Primary sclerosing cholangitis is associated with nonsmoking: a case-control study. Gastroenterology 110:1496–1502
59. Nuako KW, Ahlquist DA, Sandborn WJ et al (1998) Primary sclerosing cholangitis and colorectal carcinoma in patients with chronic ulcerative colitis: a case-control study. Cancer 82:822–826

Chapter 3
Prevention and Prognosis

Motoi Uchino, Hiroki Ikeuchi, Toshihiro Bando, Kei Hirose, Nobuyuki Hida, and Shiro Nakamura

Abstract Patients with inflammatory bowel disease (IBD) are at high risk of developing colitis-associated colorectal cancer (CA-CRC), and the risk increases with a longer disease duration and is greater in those with continuous inflammation without remission. Thus, surveillance colonoscopy is recommended for patients with IBD because of the rapid progression and extension of CA-CRC, the poor prognosis of patients diagnosed at a younger age, and the higher mortality of CA-CRC than sporadic CRC. Although the efficacy of surveillance for decreasing CA-CRC mortality remains unclear, the early detection of CA-CRC results in a survival rate of these patients similar to that of patients with ulcerative colitis (UC) who develop sporadic CRC. However, UC patients with advanced CRC have a poorer prognosis than non-UC patients with sporadic CRC. In patients with Crohn's disease, surveillance colonoscopy is difficult because of the presence of colonic strictures, such that most CRCs are diagnosed in the advanced stage and the prognosis is worse than in UC or sporadic CRC. Based on the theory of an inflammation-driven carcinogenic process as a causative factor of CA-CRC, treatment for IBD aimed at reducing inflammation may decrease the cancer risk.

Keywords Colitis-associated cancer • Prognosis • Prevention

3.1 Introduction

Patients with inflammatory bowel disease (IBD), which includes ulcerative colitis (UC) and Crohn's disease (CD), are at high risk of developing colitis-associated colorectal cancer (CA-CRC). The risk of CA-CRC increases in IBD patients with a longer duration and greater extent of colitis, continuous inflammation without remission, colitis with backwash ileitis, and primary sclerosing cholangitis [1].

The prognosis of patients with CA-CRC is generally worse than that of patients with sporadic CRC [2–4]. Surveillance colonoscopy is currently recommended by the American Gastroenterological Association, the American College of

M. Uchino (✉) • H. Ikeuchi • T. Bando • K. Hirose • N. Hida • S. Nakamura
Department of Inflammatory Bowel Disease, Hyogo College of Medicine, 1-1, Mukogawacho, Nishinomiya, Hyogo 663-8501, Japan
e-mail: uchino2s@hyo-med.ac.jp

M. Kusunoki (ed.), *Colitis-Associated Cancer*, DOI 10.1007/978-4-431-55522-3_3

Gastroenterology, the American Society for Gastrointestinal Endoscopy, and the guidelines for the management of ulcerative colitis in Japan, because patients with CA-CRC typically have a rapid disease progression and extension, a poor prognosis when diagnosed at a younger age, and a higher mortality than those with sporadic CRC [5–12]. Although the efficacy of surveillance in decreasing CA-CRC mortality is unclear, some authors have reported that the early detection of CA-CRS results in a survival rate similar to that of patients with sporadic CRC [13–15]. This chapter addresses the risk factors for CA-CRC, the prognosis of these patients, and the measures aimed at the prevention of CA-CRC.

3.2 Prognosis of Patients with UC and CA-CRC

The factors affecting the prognosis of patients with UC and CA-CRC are not well understood. The cumulative incidence of CA-CRC in UC patients is 2 % after 10 years of disease, 8 % after 20 years, and 18 % after 30 years of disease according to a meta-analysis from 2001 [1]. Previous studies identified several risk factors for CRC in UC, including longer duration and extension of colitis, concomitant primary sclerosing cholangitis, presence of pseudopolyps or backwash ileitis, and a family history of CRC [16–21]. These findings suggest that long-standing and continuous inflammation lead to carcinogenesis, resulting in CA-CRC. Recent studies have suggested that long-term failure to achieve remission from active colitis is a risk factor for CRC, whereas immunomodulators and antitumor necrosis factor were shown to be protective factors [19, 22].

Surveillance colonoscopy for CA-CRC has been largely standardized and is recognized in several guidelines as necessary in patients with long-standing colitis (>8–10 years) in the form of extended pancolitis or left-sided colitis [7–9, 11, 23, 24]. Recent studies have compared the rates of cancer detected at earlier stages (stages I–II) with the CA-CRC rates reported in previous decades [25–27]. A recent study in Japan showed that up to 75 % of CA-CRC patients examined with surveillance colonoscopy were diagnosed with early-stage CRC (stage I or 0) [15].

The first patient with CA-CRC and UC was reported in 1925 by Crohn and Rosenberg, from Mt. Sinai Hospital in New York City [28]. In 1955, before the above-cited predictors were identified and before the concept of surveillance colonoscopy was established, Sugita reported the clinical features and survival of 102 patients with CA-CRC in UC at the same institution [27]. Multiple locations of cancer, high-stage disease, tumors with a high mucin content, or cancer in a flat lesion corresponded to a poor prognosis.

The endoscopic features of CA-CRC, that is, polypoid, nodular, ulcerated, irregular raised lesions, strictures, or plaque-like lesions, resemble those of dysplasia and cancer [29]. However, a flat lesion that may not be detectable by endoscopic biopsy may harbor an underlying invasive cancer [30]. Therefore, such lesions could spread unexpectedly as an advanced cancer even with surveillance colonoscopy. The unexpected spread of cancer may also be understood based on the epidemiologic and histologic features of these tumors. Poorly differentiated, anaplastic tumors and tumors with a high mucin content are more common in CA-CRC than in sporadic CRC. CA-CRC or dysplasia may be defined as an unequivocal neoplastic alteration of the intestinal epithelium that differs from sporadic cancer [31]. CA-CRC tends to occur in multiple locations and to be of higher histologic grade than sporadic cancer [26]. In particular, there is a higher prevalence of mucinous carcinomas in CA-CRC [26, 32, 33]. A mucinous component occurs in 28 % of cases of CA-CRC [27], whereas in sporadic CRC, mucinous adenocarcinoma accounts for about 10 % of all cases [34, 35]. A recent meta-analysis suggested that mucinous adenocarcinoma has a worse prognosis than typical adenocarcinoma [34–37], although the prognosis of patients with mucinous adenocarcinoma depends on disease stage at surgery [38]. Nonetheless, the 5-year survival rate is significantly worse in patients with than without CA-CRC characterized by a mucinous component (40 % vs. 67 %; $P = 0.03$) [27]. In a comparison of CA-CRC and sporadic CRC, mucinous/signet ring cell carcinoma accounted for 17 % of the cases in CA-CRC vs. 4 % in sporadic CRC [14]. However, a large number of moderately or well-differentiated adenocarcinomas with a small tip of cancer that includes mucinous elements might be accidentally included as a typical adenocarcinoma, which has implications for the prognosis of these patients and may distort the true incidence of mucinous adenocarcinoma.

In view of the histologic findings, in 1976 Riddell et al. [39] suggested a classification that incorporates the features of dysplasia progression and which continues to be largely valid today. The authors classified dysplasia into two common types, adenomatous change and basal cell change, and into three rare types, in situ anaplasia, clear cell change, and pan-cellular change. One of the noteworthy features associated with the deeply invasive behavior of CA-CRC is the mucin component or poorly differentiated adenocarcinoma. If the tip of the tumor is involved, then the disease may extend into the lamina muscularis mucosae without rupturing this layer. Therefore, some deeply invasive CA-CRCs may go undetected during surveillance colonoscopy such that patients may unfortunately be diagnosed only when the disease has reached an advanced stage. Architectural aberrations, such as complex crypt budding, branching, or a back-to-back growth pattern, are also indicative of aggressive dysplasia and CA-CRC.

The efficacy of surveillance colonoscopy for CA-CRC has been evaluated in several studies. In an earlier review article covering the years 1980–1993, among 1916 patients who underwent surveillance colonoscopy, 92 had CA-CRC [40, 41]. Overall, 57 % of the patients were diagnosed with stage A or B disease, according to the Dukes classification, and the remainder with stage C disease. These results together with the incidental detection of CA-CRC during surgery, following barium enema, during sigmoidoscopy, or at the initial colonoscopy of a surveillance program provided strong evidence of the failure of surveillance even in patients with Dukes' A or B disease. Indeed, surveillance was considered to be successful in only 12 % of the cases. With respect to the efficacy of surveillance to detect curable stages of CA-CRC, Choi et al. [42] reported that 19 CA-CRCs (Dukes' A/B/C, 7/8/4) detected by surveillance colonoscopy were found at an earlier stage than

22 CA-CRCs detected without a surveillance program (Dukes' A/B/C, 3/6/13). Furthermore, the 5-year survival rate was higher in the patients with (77.2 %) than in those without (36.3 %) surveillance colonoscopy. Similarly, Connell et al. [43] reported a 5-year survival rate of 87 % for patients with surveillance colonoscopy, compared with 55 % for those without surveillance. In Japan, Hata et al. [13] examined the Dukes' stage of tumors in patients with and without surveillance colonoscopy and reported that four of the five CRCs found in patients undergoing surveillance were stage A, whereas three of the four CRCs in patients without surveillance were stage C. The authors concluded that surveillance is useful for detecting CA-CRC and may contribute to a better prognosis. Fujii et al. [44] analyzed the differences in the depth of cancer invasion, the incidence of lymph node and liver metastases, and the cancer stage in 41 patients with surveillance and 64 patients without surveillance. The results showed that early-stage CRC, defined as within stage T1, was more frequent in patients with than without surveillance (60.5 % vs. 27.6 %, respectively; $P = 0.004$). Patients who had undergone surveillance also had a lower incidence of lymph node metastasis than patients who did not (13.8 % vs. 52.1 %, respectively; $P = 0.002$). Finally, four of the five patients with liver metastasis and all seven of the patients with peritoneal dissemination belonged to the group without surveillance. These findings support the use of surveillance colonoscopy to improve the prognosis of CA-CRC, although surveillance cannot guarantee cancer detection at a curable stage.

With respect to the actual prognosis of CA-CRC, some studies have shown that survival is worse in patients with CA-CRC than in those with sporadic CRC, whereas according to others, survival rates are similar. Ohman et al. [45], from the Karolinska Institutet, Sweden, reported no significant difference in the 5-year survival rate between patients with CA-CRC (47 %, in 29 cases) and those with sporadic CRC (47 %, in 1032 cases). Gyde et al. [46] reported similar 5-year survival rates in a series of patients from West Midlands, England: 33.5 % in the 35 patients with CA-CRC and 32.6 % in the 462 patients with sporadic CRC. In their study from the Mayo Clinic, van Heerden et al. [47] reported that 70 patients with CA-CRC had a worse survival rate than those with sporadic CRC. They also reported that patients with CA-CRC identified incidentally during prophylactic colectomy fared well (72 % 5-year survival rate), while those with clinical symptoms or radiographic suggestion of CRC had a poor 5-year survival rate (35 %). In a report restricted to each cancer stage, Lavery et al. [48], from the Cleveland Clinic, found no significant differences in a stage-matched comparison of 79 patients with CA-CRC and sporadic CRC, although the 5-year survival rate was only 41 % in patients with CA-CRC. In a stage-matched study also from the Mayo Clinic, Delaunoit et al. [26] found similar 5-year survival rates of 53–54 % in 241 patients with CA-CRC and an equal number of those with sporadic CRC. In the recent report of Watanabe et al. [14], the 5-year overall survival rate was similar in 65 patients with CA-CRC and 62,587 patients with sporadic CRC (64.2 % vs. 68.7 %; $P = 0.58$). However, the 5-year survival rate of patients with CA-CRC when grouped according to cancer stage was significantly worse in those with stage 3 disease than in patients with sporadic CRC (43.3 % vs. 57.4 %; $P = 0.03$).

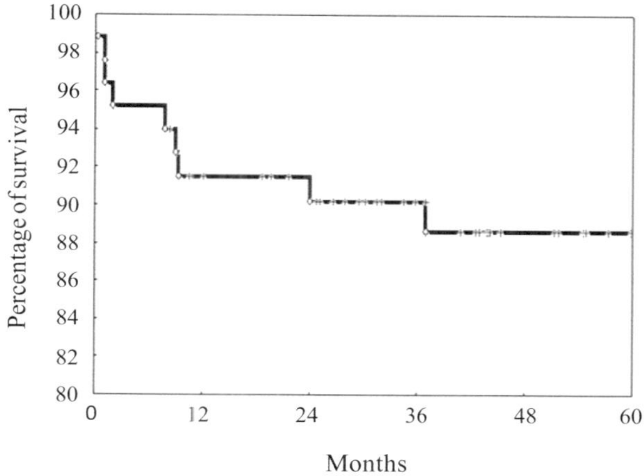

Fig. 3.1 The 5-year overall survival rate in patients with ulcerative colitis–colorectal cancer (UC-CRC). The 5-year overall survival rate was 89 % (Citation from Ref. [15])

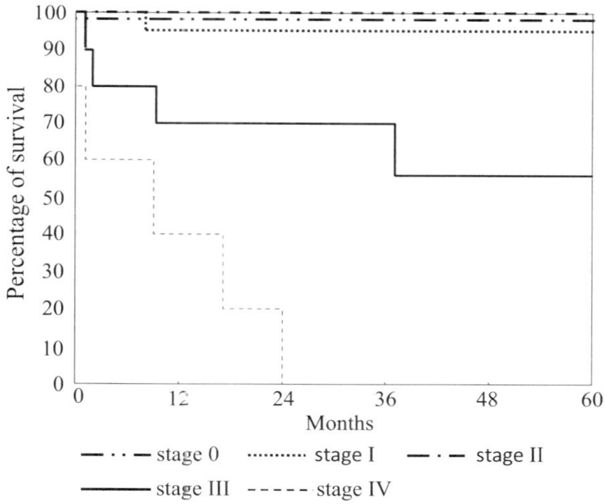

Fig. 3.2 The 5-year survival rates of patients with ulcerative colitis at each stage. Stages 0–II, 100 %; stage I, 96 %; stage III, 56 %; and stage IV, 0 % (Citation from Ref. [15])

Figures 3.1 and 3.2 provide a comparison of cases between January 1984 and December 2010 in patients with CA-CRC; the results are similar to those cited above [15]. In 83 UC patients with CA-CRC, the 5-year overall survival rate was 89 %. The actual 5-year survival rate by stage was 100 % in the 47 patients with stages 0 and II, 96 % in the 21 patients with stage I, 56 % in the ten patients with stage III, and 0 % in the five patients with stage IV [15]. Thus, the prognosis of patients with UC and CA-CRC seems to depend on cancer stage at diagnosis and the pathological features of the tumor.

3.3 Prognosis of Patients with CD and CA-CRC

Unlike in UC, the risk and prognosis of CA-CRC in CD patients are less well validated. Previous studies on the risk of intestinal cancer in CD reported inconsistent results, with relative risk estimates ranging from 0.8 to 20.0 [49]. Previous studies concluded that the predictors of CA-CRC in CD must be evaluated based on the intestinal segment(s) involved by CD, given the different disease behaviors and thus the potential for cancer in the small bowel, colorectal, or anal region.

The risk of CRC in long-standing CD involving the colon is probably comparable to that of UC [2, 3, 50–55]. In a Danish nationwide cohort study, although the relative risk (RR) of CRC in IBD was low in the first years after diagnosis, it was significantly higher than in the background population after a disease duration of 13 years, reaching 50 % [56]. These results are also consistent with the current surveillance guidelines of the American Gastroenterological Association [5] and the British Society for Gastroenterology [57], both of which recommend the initiation of surveillance after 8–10 years of disease duration for CD, as for extensive UC. However, up to a third of IBD patients develop CRC prior to the initial surveillance colonoscopy [56, 58, 59], suggesting the need to reconsider the present surveillance strategy. An additional complicating factor is that the majority of patients with extended colonic CD lesions may require colectomy after a shorter disease duration than is the case in UC patients.

A meta-analysis from 2005 by Jess et al. [60] limited to population-based studies estimated a pooled overall standardized incidence ratio (SIR) for CRC in CD patients of 1.9 [95 % confidence interval (CI), 1.4–2.5]. Separate risk estimates for cancer in the colon and rectum resulted in a significantly higher risk for colon cancer (SIR = 2.5; 95 % CI, 1.7–3.5), while there was no significantly increased pooled risk for rectal cancer (SIR = 1.4; 95 % CI, 0.8–2.6). The risk of CRC was significantly higher in CD patients with colonic involvement (SIR = 4.3; 95 % CI, 2.0–9.4).

The incidence of CRC in CD is similar in Japan and Western countries, but the anatomic location of CRC differs between the respective populations. The study of Jess et al. [60] included populations from North America, Scandinavia, and Israel. Yano et al. [61] found that the SIR for CRC in Japanese patients with CD was 2.79 (95 % CI, 1.28–5.29); in that series, eight of nine patients with CD and CRC had anorectal cancer (ARC). Mizushima et al. [62] also found that the risk of CRC was significantly higher in patients with CD than in the general population (SIR = 5.80; 95 % CI, 2.13–12.68); in their series, five of six patients with CD had ARC. In a review of the Japanese literature, Sugita et al. [63] reported a high incidence (55–89 %) of ARC in patients with CD and CRC. A noteworthy feature of that study was the finding that 55–68 % of the ARC cases involved a colonic stricture without a fistula. In CD, ARC can arise at a similar (or higher) rate in patients with strictures as in those with fistulas. The anatomic location of CRC in CD patients may show racial differences, as suggested by the higher incidence of colonic involvement in Western countries and a higher incidence of anorectal involvement in Asian countries.

With respect to ARC in CD, despite the lack of population-based studies specifically evaluating ARC and although previous studies were from Western countries, it seems that malignancy rarely arises in perianal fistulas [64, 65], but cancer can certainly arise from a long-standing perianal CD fistula [66–68]. Iesalnieks et al. [69] reviewed 23 published reports describing 59 CD patients with adenocarcinoma arising from perianal fistulas. The authors noted that, while the exact pathogenesis of ARC is unclear, the risk of malignant transformation is significantly higher in patients with fistulizing inflammation. They also observed that adenocarcinomas associated with anal fistulas in patients without CD seem to share many features of ARC in those with CD, including a long-term history of perianal fistula (10–20 years) and an increased incidence of mucin-producing adenocarcinomas. Thus, the presence of a long-standing fistula, rather than the disease behaviors of CD itself, seems to be an important predisposing factor for ARC.

Cancer surveillance can be difficult in patients with CD regardless of the anatomic location of either CRC or ARC, because the thoroughness of the examination may be limited by the presence of strictures. Ky et al. [68] suggested that, especially in ARC, carcinoma arising in a CD fistula is very difficult to diagnose, because the examination for anorectal lesions may be limited by pain, stricture, or induration of the perianal and perineal tissues. They noted that although examination under anesthesia can also overlook the lesion, it generally increases the yield of biopsies or curettage of the fistulous tracts. Examination under anesthesia in these cases is also recommended in Japan, but its efficacy has yet to be confirmed [63].

Regardless of differences in the anatomic locations of CRC in different populations, the prognosis of CRC is worse in CD patients than in UC patients. A nationwide population-based cohort study in Denmark [70] established that CD patients with CRC had a significantly worse mortality. Of patients with a history of CD, 62 % died within the first 5 years compared with 56 % of the matched cohort consisting of patients with CRC but without IBD. For CRC patients with CD, the corresponding mortality ratios compared with patients with non-IBD CRC were 1.33 (95 % CI, 1.06–1.66) and 1.26 (95 % CI, 1.07–1.49).

The prognosis of patients with CD and ARC is poor. Igors et al. [69] reported the survival data of 59 CD patients with ARC. The overall survival rates after proctectomy were 88 % at 1 year, 54 % at 3 years, and 26 % at 5 years. Perirectal lymph node metastases were significantly associated with poor outcome ($P < 0.0001$), and all patients with lymph node metastases ($n = 15$) died within 40 months after proctectomy. In a review of the Japanese literature, the overall survival rate after proctectomy was similar: 45 % at 5 years and 30 % at 10 years, even in patients who received postoperative chemotherapy. The overall 5-year survival rate of CA-CRC in 32 patients with CD at our institution between January 1984 and April 2014 was 39.3 % (Fig. 3.3). The patients included three with stage I, 16 with stage II, and six with stage III disease as well as seven patients with an unclassified advanced stage of cancer.

Small bowel carcinoma (SBC) in patients with CD has been discussed controversially. SBC in patients with small bowel CD has long been viewed as a rare and

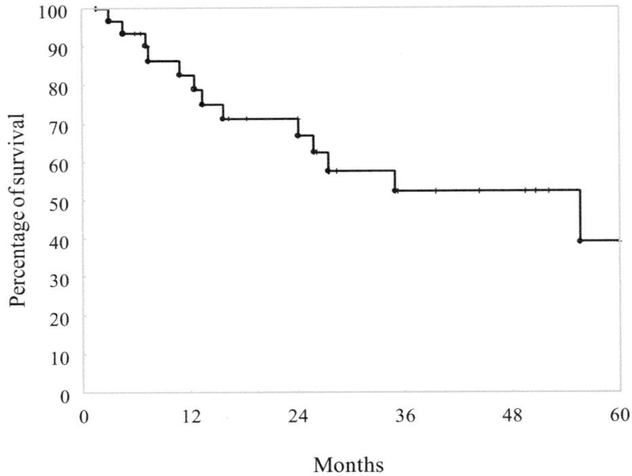

Fig. 3.3 The 5-year overall survival rate of intestinal cancer in patients with Crohn's disease. The overall 5-year survival rate in 32 patients was 39.3 % (Unpublished data at our institution)

ominous disease for which any form of screening or early detection strategy is unlikely to be useful [49]. A meta-analysis from 2005 by Jess et al. [60] found that, although the pooled overall SIR for CRC in CD patients was 1.9 (95 % CI, 1.4–2.5), the SIRs of SBC were not increased either in patients with ileocolonic CD (SIR = 2.6; 95 % CI, 0.8–8.2) or in those with pure jejunoileal disease (SIR = 0.9; 95 % CI, 0.2–4.1). In the meta-analysis of Canavan et al. [49], also published in 2005, analyses of site-specific CD showed no increase in the RR of SBC in the subset of CD patients with ileal disease (RR = 1.1; 95 % CI, 0.8–1.5).

In five previous population-based meta-analyses, the SIR of SBC ranged from 18.75 to 33.2 in patients with CD [49, 60, 70–72]. Jess et al. [60] found that the number of cases of SBC in patients with CD of the small bowel (nine in 26,780 patient-years) was similar to that of CRC in patients with CD of the colon (ten in 32,833 patient-years). In another report based on a hospital cohort of 1935 patients with CD involving the small bowel [73], the cumulative risk of SBC in CD was estimated to be 2 (95 % CI, 0–8) and 22 (95 % CI, 7–64) per 1000 patients after 10 and 25 years of follow-up, respectively. In a recent large, prospective, cohort study of SBC in CD [74], five SBCs were found in 8222 patients with small bowel CD (either alone or associated with colonic CD) during a median follow-up of 35 months (range, 29–40 months). The incidence rates of SBC were 0.235 per 1000 patient-years (95 % CI, 0.076–0.547) among patients with small bowel CD and 0.464 per 1000 patient-years (95 % CI, 0.127–1.190) among those with small bowel CD for 8 years. This accounted for approximately 30 % of the risk of CRC in patients with CD of the colon. Patients with small bowel CD and small bowel CD for 8 years had an SBC SIR of 34.9 (95 % CI, 11.3–81.5) and 46.0 (95 % CI, 12.5–117.8), respectively.

Dossett et al. [75] summarized the features of 154 cases of SBC in CD reported in Europe and America. SBC occurred more frequently in males than in females (M:F = 2.4:1). The age at diagnosis ranged from 21 to 86 years (mean age,

51.3 years), and the average duration of CD was 24.5 years (range, 0–45 years) [75]. CD patients who developed SBC were younger than those with de novo cancers, which occurred mainly in patients 60–69 years of age [76, 77]. Ileal tumors occurred at a rate of 75 %. The presence of tumor in previously bypassed segments of the intestine was 20.3 %. Obstruction was the most common manifestation (76 %), whereas hemorrhage, fistula, and perforation were present in 3.9 %, 3.9 %, and 5.4 % of the cases, respectively. The majority of the diagnoses were made at the time of surgery (35.4 %) or postoperatively (61.5 %). Only 3.1 % of the cases were diagnosed preoperatively.

Thus, patients with CD are also at risk of CA-SBC, albeit the incidence is lower than that of CRC or ARC. However, while the incidence of SBC is low in the general population, it is significantly higher in patients with CD (RR = 27) [78]. Nonetheless, since <1 % of patients with CD will develop SBC and given the similarity of SBC findings and those of CD lesions on some examinations, the diagnosis of SBC in CD patients can be very challenging [79, 80]. Moreover, the prognosis of CD patients with SBC is poor. In the study of Elriz et al. [74], four of the five patients with SBC, diagnosed at an advanced stage by resected specimens, died within 3 years. In the study of Dossett et al. [75], based on 154 cases of SBC in CD reported in Europe and America, the survival rates after 1 and 2 years were 49.6 % and 27 %, respectively. Even in SBC in patients with non-CD, diagnosis was made at a late stage because of limited and insensitive examinations or vague presenting symptoms. Consequently, these patients have a worse prognosis, with a reported 5-year survival of 26 % [81, 82].

In all reports on the incidence of CRC, patients with CD were diagnosed with a more advanced stage of disease than those with UC or no IBD: either Dukes' B or C; stage 3, with lymph node involvement; stage 4; or T2 or T3 with a positive N number [5, 56–59]. Furthermore, in CD, tumors with mucinous components or poorly differentiated adenocarcinomas are not uncommon, even in CA-CRC in CD, regardless of the site of anatomic involvement [26]. In conclusion, the prognosis of CA-CRC in patients with CD may depend on the cancer stage at diagnosis and the pathological features, as in UC; but in patients with long-standing CD, the possibility of concomitant cancer should be considered even in sites of strictureplasty [82–84].

3.4 Chemoprevention of CAC

The results of studies on the risk factors CA-CRC [16–21] suggest that long-standing and continuous inflammation lead to carcinogenesis and in turn CA-CRC. It is also clear that long-term failure to achieve remission from active colitis is a risk factor for CA-CRC [19, 22]. Chronic inflammation may contribute to carcinogenesis by generating a favorable microenvironment for cancer development and progression. Increased concentrations of inflammatory cytokines or mediators, such as reactive oxygen and nitrogen species or cyclooxygenase-2-associated prostaglandins, and alterations of DNA, RNA, proteins, or lipids have been invoked as events leading to tumor formation. For example, the p53 tumor suppressor gene is mutated in the inflamed mucosa, and expression of the gene was shown to correlate with the intensity of inflammation and with the degree of dysplasia [85]. Thus, it may be that strategies aimed at reducing the inflammation in IBD may also decrease the risk of CA-CRC. Several approaches to achieving this goal are described in the following.

3.4.1 Probiotics

The human gut microflora, comprising some 100 trillion microbial organisms, is critical in maintaining host health, both in the gastrointestinal tract itself and systemically, through the absorption of metabolites [86]. Recent studies have implicated specific strains of bacteria in the regulation of intestinal homeostasis, by delivering regulatory signals to the epithelium, to the mucosal immune system, and to the neuromuscular activity of the gut [87, 88]. However, some commensal and pathogenic organisms belonging to the human enteric microbiome contribute to the pathogenesis of IBD and CRC. Therefore, the use of probiotic bacteria to manipulate gut bacterial composition and local metabolite production has been explored as a therapeutic intervention to prevent CRC. Probiotics are live microbial food supplements with positive effects on host health. However, the efficacy of probiotics in this setting is unclear, and studies in mice have yielded controversial results [88–90]. To date, there have been no proper evaluations in humans.

3.4.2 Aminosalicylate

Patients with IBD are commonly administered 5-aminosalicylate (5-ASA) as maintenance therapy, which in in vitro studies was shown to have antineoplastic properties by inhibiting the nuclear kappa-B pathway involved in tumor progression [91]. However, the evidence for a potential chemoprophylactic effect of 5-ASA is contradictory. In 2005, Velayos et al. [92] reported a meta-analysis of nine studies examining the effect of 5-ASA in preventing CA-CRC in IBD. The pooled analysis revealed a protective effect of 5-ASA use on the risk of CA-CRC (odds ratio = 0.51; 95 % CI, 0.37–0.69). However, a chemopreventive effect of 5-ASA has not been confirmed in case–control and population-based studies [93–95]. In a recent meta-analysis, Nguyen et al. [96] reported a pooled adjusted odds ratio of 0.95 (95 % CI, 0.66–1.38) for CA-CRC in patients with IBD treated with 5-ASA, nor did 5-ASA seem to have a protective effect in preventing CA-CRC in IBD. However, long-standing mild colitis, which could be maintained by 5-ASA administration alone, without aggressive therapy such as corticosteroids, immunomodulators, or biologics, could increase the risk of CA-CRC [15], by maintaining a state of chronic inflammation without complete remission or mucosal healing.

3.4.3 Immunomodulators

An increasing number of IBD patients are being treated with the thiopurine drugs azathioprine and 6-mercaptopurine, based on the consideration that aggressive therapy can induce complete remission and may therefore have a preventive effect. However, data on the potential chemopreventive effect of thiopurines in IBD are conflicting. In the CESAME study [58], nearly half of the 19,484 IBD patients had been exposed to thiopurines; among current users, the adjusted hazard ratio (HR) for CA-CRC was 0.57 (95 % CI, 0.24–1.32), thus ruling out a significant protective effect of thiopurine use on CA-CRC risk in the general IBD population. However, in a subanalysis confined to IBD patients with long-standing extensive colitis, current treatment with thiopurines reduced the risk of advanced CRC significantly (HR 0.28; 95 % CI, 0.09–0.89). In a Dutch cohort study, van Schaik et al. [97] estimated the effect of thiopurines on the risk of CA-CRC in an IBD cohort of 2578 IBD patients, of whom 770 had been exposed to thiopurines. They found that thiopurine exposure decreased the risk of advanced CA-CRC significantly (adjusted HR = 0.10; 95 % CI, 0.01–0.75). However, in a Danish, nationwide, population-based study, Pasternak et al. [98] found no effect of thiopurine on the occurrence of CA-CRC among 43,969 IBD patients, of whom 12 % had been exposed to thiopurines (adjusted RR = 1.00; 95 % CI, 0.61–1.63). Similar results were reported in another large population-based study from the United Kingdom [99].

3.4.4 Biologics

Recent data from models of experimental colitis have demonstrated the tumor-promoting effect of tumor necrosis factor (TNF)-α [100]; but, only a few studies have evaluated the effect of new biological treatments, such as anti-TNF-α, on the risk of CA-CRC, as they have not been used long enough relative to the latency of CA-CRC. In a Dutch nested case–control study, Baars et al. [22] evaluated the risk factors for CA-CRC by comparing 173 CA-CRC patients with 393 non-CRC patients with IBD. They found that the use of anti-TNF-α was a protective factor for the development of CA-CRC (odds ratio = 0.09; 95 % CI, 0.01–0.68). In a Danish nationwide population-based cohort study, the risk of CA-CRC was compared between patients treated or not with anti-TNF-α. There was no correlation between anti-TNF-α and the prevalence of CA-CRC (adjusted RR = 1.06; 95 % CI, 0.33–3.40) [101]. Given that anti-TNF-α may be both tumor promoting and tumor preventing, further studies are needed to confirm its efficacy as a chemopreventive agent.

3.5 Prophylactic Efficacy of Proctocolectomy

3.5.1 Proctocolectomy in Patients with UC

Surveillance colonoscopy for CA-CRC has been standardized, and its use in patients with long-standing IBD ($\geq$8–10 years) has been widely advocated [7–9, 11, 23, 24]. Dysplasia or cancer found in surveillance is an absolute indication for proctocolectomy in patients with UC. Although it remains unclear whether proctocolectomy can decrease the incidence of CA-CRC in UC and improve the prognosis of these patients, the 5-year survival rate was higher in patients who underwent surveillance (87 %) than in those who did not (55 %) [43]. In Japan, Hata et al. [13] suggested that surveillance would allow the detection of CA-CRC at an earlier stage. In a recent review and meta-analysis of the incidence of CA-CRC, the risk of UC patients developing CRC was found to have decreased steadily over the last six decades [102]. Whether these improvements can be attributed to surveillance colonoscopy and prophylactic proctocolectomy remains to be determined.

3.5.2 Proctocolectomy in Patients with Anorectal CD

In patients at risk of SBC, prophylactic resection of the small intestine is contraindicated by its absolute necessity for nutrient absorption, although total parenteral nutrition therapy can be considered. However, in patients with anorectal CD, prophylactic proctectomy may decrease the incidence of ARC. As discussed in Sect. 3.3, ARC is rarely detected in its early stage owing to the difficulty of proper surveillance and accurate diagnosis. Furthermore, ostomy diversion of anorectal CD increases the risk of ARC [64, 65, 69]. However, in patients with severe perianal disease with stricture, in whom both medical management and local surgical treatment have failed, the first surgical option is a diverting colostomy or ileostomy. If these do not provide sufficient relief, the final option is proctectomy, performed in 10–20 % of patients with perianal CD [103, 104]. Proctectomy generally consists of either a low Hartmann's procedure or a complete proctectomy with sphincter resection. The disadvantages of Hartmann's procedure include the risk of ARC in the residual distal rectum. This can cause persisting complaints of Crohn's disease, and anastomotic breakdown will result in a presacral abscess draining and fistulizing through the perineum [105–108]. Therefore, in our institution, complete proctectomy is preferred when the stricturing anorectal lesion, regardless of the presence of a fistula tract, cannot be improved by any treatment. In our experience, proctectomy for these lesions improves not only the severe symptoms of anorectal lesions but also the incidence of ARC. However, an as yet unresolved problem is that the perineal wound after proctocolectomy heals poorly and there is a high incidence of persistent sinus in patients with CD [109, 110]. Long-term cohort studies, performed after several decades, are still needed to determine the outcomes of these patients.

References

1. Eaden JA, Abrams KR, Mayberry JF (2001) The risk of colorectal cancer in ulcerative colitis: a meta-analysis. Gut 48:526–535
2. Softley A, Clamp SE, Watkinson G et al (1988) The natural history of inflammatory bowel disease: has there been change in the last 20 years? Scand J Gastroenterol Suppl 144:20
3. Richards ME, Rickert RR, Nance FC (1989) Crohn's disease-associated carcinoma. A poorly recognized complication of inflammatory bowel disease. Ann Surg 209:764
4. Peyrin-Biroulet L, Lepage C, Jooste V et al (2012) Colorectal cancer in inflammatory bowel diseases: a population-based study (1976–2008). Inflamm Bowel Dis 18:2247–2251
5. Farraye FA, Odze RD, Eaden J et al (2010) AGA medical position statement on the diagnosis and management of colorectal neoplasia in inflammatory bowel disease. Gastroenterology 138:738
6. Winawer S, Fletcher R, Rex D et al (2003) Colorectal cancer screening and surveillance: clinical guidelines and rationale-Update based on new evidence. Gastroenterology 124:544
7. Kornbluth A, Sachar DB (1997) Ulcerative colitis practice guidelines in adults. American College of Gastroenterology, Practice Parameters Committee. Am J Gastroenterol 92:204
8. Leighton JA, Shen B, Baron TH et al (2006) ASGE guideline: endoscopy in the diagnosis and treatment of inflammatory bowel disease. Gastrointest Endosc 63:558
9. Eaden JA, Mayberry JF (2002) British Society for Gastroenterology, Association of Coloproctology for Great Britain and Ireland. Guidelines for screening and surveillance of asymptomatic colorectal cancer in patients with inflammatory bowel disease. Gut 51:V10
10. Carins SR, Scholefield JH, Steele RJ et al (2010) Guidelines for colorectal cancer screening and surveillance in moderate and high risk groups (update from2002). Gut 59:666
11. Hibi T, Ueno F (2010) Guidelines for the management of ulcerative colitis in Japan – Developed through integration of evidence and consensus among experts – Research Group for Intractable Inflammatory Bowel Disease 2006. Research on Intractable Diseases, Health and Labour Sciences. Research Grants from the Ministry of Health, Labour and Welfare, Japan. IBD Res 4:189–239
12. Rutter MD, Saunders PP, Wilkinson KH et al (2006) Thirty years analysis of colonoscopic surveillance program for neoplasia in ulcerative colitis. Gastroenterology 130:1030–1038
13. Hata K, Watanabe T, Kazama S et al (2003) Earlier surveillance colonoscopy programme improves survival in patients with ulcerative colitis associated colorectal cancer: results of a 23-year surveillance programme in the Japanese population. Br J Cancer 89:1232–1236
14. Watanabe T, Konishi T, Kishimoto J et al (2011) Ulcerative colitis-associated colorectal cancer shows a poorer survival than sporadic colorectal cancer: a nationwide Japanese study. Inflamm Bowel Dis 17:802–808
15. Matsuoka H, Ikeuchi H, Uchino M et al (2013) Clinicopathological features of ulcerative colitis-associated colorectal cancer pointing to efficiency of surveillance colonoscopy in a large retrospective Japanese cohort. Int J Color Dis 28:829–834
16. Ekbom A, Helmick C, Zack M et al (1990) Ulcerative colitis and colorectal cancer. A population-based study. N Engl J Med 323:1228–1233
17. Broome U, Lofberg R, Veress B et al (1995) Primary sclerosing cholangitis and ulcerative colitis: evidence for increased neoplastic potential. Hepatology 22:1404–1408
18. Askling J, Dickman PW, Karlen P et al (2001) Family history as a risk factor for colorectal cancer in inflammatory bowel disease. Gastroenterology 120:1356–1362
19. Rutter M, Saunders B, Wilkinson K et al (2004) Severity of inflammation is a risk factor for colorectal neoplasia in ulcerative colitis. Gastroenterology 125:451–459
20. Rutter MD, Saunders BP, Wilkinson KH et al (2004) Cancer surveillance in long-standing ulcerative colitis: endoscopic appearances help predict cancer risk. Gut 53:1813–1816
21. Velayos FS, Loftus EV Jr, Jess T et al (2006) Predictive and protective factors associated with colorectal cancer in ulcerative colitis: a case-control study. Gastroenterology 130:1941–1949

22. Baars JE, Looman CW, Steyerberg EW et al (2011) The risk of inflammatory bowel disease-related colorectal carcinoma is limited: Results from a nationwide nested case-control study. Am J Gastroenterol 106:319–328
23. Ooi CJ, Fock KM, Makharia GK et al (2010) The Asia-Pacific consensus on ulcerative colitis. J Gastroenterol Hepatol 25:453–468
24. Hida N, Nakamura S, Hahm KB et al (2014) A questionnaire-based survey on the diagnosis and management of inflammatory bowel disease in East Asian countries in 2012. Digestion 89:88–103
25. Harpaz N, Talbot IC (1996) Colorectal cancer in idiopathic inflammatory bowel disease. Semin Diagn Pathol 13:339–357
26. Delaunoit T, Limburg PJ, Goldberg RM et al (2006) Colorectal cancer prognosis among patients with inflammatory bowel disease. Clin Gastroenterol Hepatol 4:335–342
27. Sugita A, Greenstein AJ, Ribeiro MB et al (1993) Survival with colorectal cancer in ulcerative colitis. A study of 102 cases. Ann Surg 218:189–195
28. Crohn BB, Rosenberg H (1925) The sigmoidoscopic picture of chronic ulcerative colitis (nonspecific). Am J Med Sci 170:220–228
29. Butt JH, Konishi F, Morson BC et al (1983) Macroscopic lesions in dysplasia and carcinoma complicating ulcerative colitis. Dig Dis Sci 28:18
30. Blackstone MO, Riddell RH, Rogers BH et al (1981) Dysplasia-associated lesion or mass (DALM) detected by colonoscopy in long-standing ulcerative colitis: an indication for colectomy. Gastroenterology 80:366
31. Riddell RH, Goldman H, Ransohoff DF et al (1983) Dysplasia in inflammatory bowel disease: standardized classification with provisional clinical applications. Hum Pathol 14:931–968
32. Fogt F, Vortmeyer AO, Goldman H et al (1998) Comparison of genetic alterations in colonic adenoma and ulcerative colitis-associated dysplasia and carcinoma. Hum Pathol 29:131–136
33. Nugent FW, Haggit RC, Colcher H, Kutteruf GC et al (1979) Malignant potential of chronic ulcerative colitis Preliminary report. Gastroenterology 76:1–5
34. Verhulst J, Ferdinande L, Demetter P et al (2012) Mucinous subtype as prognostic factor in colorectal cancer: a systematic review and meta-analysis. J Clin Pathol 65:381–388
35. Hyngstrom JR, Hu CY, Xing Y et al (2012) Clinicopathology and outcomes for mucinous and signet-ring colorectal carcinoma: analysis from the National Cancer Data Base. Ann Surg Oncol 19:2814–2821
36. Chew MH, Yeo SA, Ng ZP et al (2010) Critical analysis of mucin and signet ring cell as prognostic factors in an Asian population of 2,764 sporadic colorectal cancers. Int J Color Dis 25:1221–1229
37. Chen JX, Tang XD, Xiang DB et al (2012) TNM stages and prognostic features of colorectal mucinous adenocarcinomas: a meta analysis. Asian Pac J Cancer Prev 13:3427–3430
38. Nitsche U, Zimmermann A, Spath C et al (2013) Mucinous and signet-ring cell colorectal cancers differ from classical adenocarcinomas in tumor biology and prognosis. Ann Surg 258:775–783
39. Riddell RH (1976) The precarcinomatous phase of ulcerative colitis. Curr Top Pathol 63:179–219
40. Axon AT (1994) Cancer surveillance in ulcerative colitis – a time for reappraisal. Gut 35:587–589
41. Lynch DA, Lobo AJ, Sobala GM, Dixon MF, Axon AT et al (1993) Failure of colonoscopic surveillance in ulcerative colitis. Gut 34:1075–1080
42. Choi PM, Nugent FW, Schoetz DJ Jr et al (1993) Colonoscopic surveillance reduces mortality from colorectal cancer in ulcerative colitis. Gastroenterology 105:418–424
43. Connell WR, Lennard-Jones JE, Williams CB et al (1994) Factors affecting the outcome of endoscopic surveillance for cancer in ulcerative colitis. Gastroenterology 107:934–944
44. Fujii S, Fujimori T, Chiba T et al (2003) Efficacy of surveillance and molecular markers for detection of ulcerative colitis-associated colorectal neoplasia. J Gastroenterol 38:1117–1125

45. Ohman U (1982) Colorectal carcinoma in patients with ulcerative colitis. Am J Surg 144:344–349
46. Gyde SN, Prior P, Thompson H et al (1984) Survival of patients with colorectal cancer complicating ulcerative colitis. Gut 25:228–231
47. van Heerden JA, Beart RW Jr (1980) Carcinoma of the colon and rectum complicating chronic ulcerative colitis. Dis Colon Rectum 23:155–159
48. Lavery IC, Chiulli RA, Jagelman DG et al (1982) Survival with carcinoma arising in mucosal ulcerative colitis. Ann Surg 195:508–512
49. Canavan C, Abrams KR, Mayberry J (2006) Meta-analysis: colorectal and small bowel cancer risk in patients with Crohn's disease. Aliment Pharmacol Ther 23:1097–1104
50. Weedon DD, Shorter RG, Ilstrup DM et al (1973) Crohn's disease and cancer. N Engl J Med 289:1099
51. Ekbom A, Heimick C, Zack M et al (1990) Increased risk of large-bowel cancer in Crohn's disease with colonic involvement. Lancet 336:357
52. Rubio CA, Befrits R (1997) Colorectal adenocarcinoma in Crohn's disease: a retrospective histologic study. Dis Colon Rectum 40:1072
53. Friedman S, Rubin PH, Bodian C et al (2001) Screening and surveillance colonoscopy in chronic Crohn's colitis. Gastroenterology 120:820
54. Maykel JA, Hagerman G, Mellgren AF et al (2006) Crohn's colitis: the incidence of dysplasia and adenocarcinoma in surgical patients. Dis Colon Rectum 49:950
55. Moreels TG, Pelckmans PA (2008) Double-balloon endoscope for failed conventional colonoscopy. Clin Gastroenterol Hepatol 6:259
56. Jess T, Simonsen J, Jørgensen KT et al (2012) Decreasing risk of colorectal cancer in patients with inflammatory bowel disease over 30 years. Gastroenterology 143:375–381
57. Cairns SR, Scholefield JH, Steele RJ et al (2010) Guidelines for colorectal cancer screening and surveillance in moderate and high risk groups (update from 2002). Gut 59:666–689
58. Beaugerie L, Svrcek M, Seksik P et al (2013) Risk of colorectal high-grade dysplasia and cancer in a prospective observational cohort of patients with inflammatory bowel disease. Gastroenterology 145:166–175
59. Baars JE, Kuipers EJ, van Haastert M et al (2012) Age at diagnosis of inflammatory bowel disease influences early development of colorectal cancer in inflammatory bowel disease patients: a nationwide, long-term survey. J Gastroenterol 47:1308–1322
60. Jess T, Gamborg M, Matzen P et al (2005) Increased risk of intestinal cancer in Crohn's disease: a meta-analysis of population-based cohort studies. Am J Gastroenterol 100:2724–2729
61. Yano Y, Matsui T, Hirai F et al (2013) Cancer risk in Japanese Crohn's disease patients: investigation of the standardized incidence ratio. J Gastroenterol Hepatol 28:1300–1305
62. Mizushima T, Ohno Y, Nakajima K et al (2010) Malignancy in Crohn's disease: incidence and clinical characteristics in Japan. Digestion 81:265–270
63. Sugita A, Koganei K, Tatsumi K et al (2013) Management of rectal cancer including cancer in the anal fistula with Crohn's disease. Nihon Shokakibyo Gakkai Zasshi 110:396–402
64. Smith R, Hicks D, Tomljanovich PI et al (2008) Adenocarcinoma arising from chronic perianal Crohn's disease: case report and review of the literature. Am Surg 74:59–61
65. Ky A, Sohn N, Weinstein MA et al (2010) Carcinoma arising in anorectal fistulas of Crohn's disease. Dis Colon Rectum 41:992–996
66. Iesalnieks I, Gaertner WB, Glass H et al (2010) Fistula-associated anal adenocarcinoma in Crohn's disease. Inflamm Bowel Dis 16:1643–1648
67. Barrs JE, Kulpers EJ, Dijkstra G et al (201) Malignant transformation of perianal and enterocutaneous fistulas is rare: results of 17 years of follow-up from The Netherlands. Scand J Gastroenterol 46:319–325
68. Ky A, Sohn N, Weinstein MA et al (1998) Carcinoma arising in anorectal fistulas of Crohn's disease. Dis Colon Rectum 41:992–996

69. Igors I, Wolfgang B, Heidi G et al (2010) Fistula-associated anal adenocarcinoma in Crohn's disease. Inflamm Bowel Dis 16:1643–1648
70. Ording AG (2013) Five-Year Mortality in Colorectal Cancer Patients with Ulcerative Colitis or Crohn's Disease: A Nationwide Population-based Cohort Study. Inflamm Bowel Dis 19:800–805
71. Laukoetter MG, Mennigen R, Hannig CM et al (2011) Intestinal cancer risk in Crohn's disease: a meta-analysis. J Gastrointest Surg 15:576–583
72. Von Roon AC, Reese G, Teare J et al (2007) The risk of cancer in patients with Crohn's disease. Dis Colon Rectum 50:839–855
73. Palascak-Juif V, Bouvier AM, Cones J et al (2005) Small bowel adenocarcinoma in patients with Crohn's disease compared with small bowel adenocarcinoma de novo. Inflamm Bowel Dis 11:828–832
74. Elriz K, Carrat F, Carbonnel F et al (2013) Incidence, Presentation, and Prognosis of Small Bowel Adenocarcinoma in Patients with Small Bowel Crohn's Disease: A Prospective Observational Study. Inflamm Bowel Dis 19:1823–1826
75. Dossett LA, White LM, Welch DC et al (2007) Small bowel adenocarcinoma complicating Crohn's disease: case series and review of the literature. Am Surg 73:1181–1187
76. Solem CA, Harmsen WS, Zinsmeister AR et al (2004) Small intestinal adenocarcinoma in Crohn's disease: a case-control study. Inflamm Bowel Dis 10:32–35
77. Negri E, Bosetti C, La Vecchia C et al (1999) Risk factors for adenocarcinoma of the small intestine. Int J Cancer 82:171–174
78. Kamiya T, Ando T, Ishiguro K et al (2012) Intestinal cancers occurring in patients with Crohn's disease. J Gastroenterol Hepatol 27:103–107
79. Michelassi F, Testa G, Pomidor WJ et al (1993) Adenocarcinoma complicating Crohn's disease. Dis Colon Rectum 36:654–661
80. Higashi D, Futami K, Kojima D et al (2012) Cancer of the small intestine in patients with Crohn's disease. Anticancer Res 33:2977–2980
81. Gill SS, Heuman DM, Mihas AA (2001) Small intestinal neoplasia. J Clin Gastroenterol 33:267–282
82. Halfdanarson TR, McWilliams RR, Donohue JH et al (2010) A single-institution experience with 491 cases of small bowel adenocarcinoma. Am J Surg 199:797–803
83. Jaskowiak NT, Michelassi F (2001) Adenocarcinoma at a strictureplasty site in Crohn's disease: report of a case. Dis Colon Rectum 44:284–287
84. Partridge SK, Hodin RA (2004) Small bowel adenocarcinoma at a strictureplasty site in a patients with Crohn's disease: report of a case. Dis Colon Rectum 47:778–781
85. Laurent C, Svrcek M, Flejou JF et al (2011) Immunohistochemical expression of CDX2, beta-catenin and TP53 in inflammatory bowel disease-associated colorectal cancer. Inflamm Bowel Dis 17:232–240
86. Moore WE, Holdeman LV (1974) Human fecal flora: the normal flora of 20 Japanese-Hawaiians. Appl Microbiol 27:961–979
87. Shanahan F (2004) Probiotics in inflammatory bowel disease–therapeutic rationale and role. Adv Drug Deliv Rev 56:809–818
88. Tuohy KM, Rouzaud GC, Bruck WM et al (2005) Modulation of the human gut microflora towards improved health using prebiotics–assessment of efficacy. Curr Pharm Des 11:75–90
89. Bassaganya-Riera J, Viladomiu M, Pedragosa M et al (2012) Immunoregulatory mechanisms underlying prevention of colitis-associated colorectal cancer by probiotic bacteria. PLoS ONE 7, e34676. doi:10.1371/journal pone.0034676
90. Arthur JC, Gharaibeh RZ, Uronis JM et al (2013) VSL#3 probiotic modifies mucosal microbial composition but does not reduce colitis-associated colorectal cancer. Sci Rep 3:2868. doi:10.1038/srep02868
91. Kaiser GC, Yan F, Polk DB (1999) Mesalamine blocks tumor necrosis factor growth inhibition and nuclear factor kappaB activation in mouse colonocytes. Gastroenterology 116:602–609

92. Velayos FS, Terdiman JP, Walsh JM (2005) Effect of 5-aminosalicylate use on colorectal cancer and dysplasia risk: a systematic review and metaanalysis of observational studies. Am J Gastroenterol 100:1345–1353
93. Bernstein CN, Nugent Z, Blanchard JF (2011) 5-aminosalicylate is not chemoprophylactic for colorectal cancer in IBD: a population based study. Am J Gastroenterol 106:731–736
94. Jess T, Loftus EV, Velayos FS et al (2007) Risk factors for colorectal neoplasia in inflammatory bowel disease: a nested case-control study from Copenhagen county, Denmark and Olmsted county, Minnesota. Am J Gastroenterol 102:829–836
95. Terdiman JP, Steinbuch M, Blumentals WA et al (2007) 5-Aminosalicylic acid therapy and the risk of colorectal cancer among patients with inflammatory bowel disease. Inflamm Bowel Dis 13:367–371
96. Nguyen GC, Gulamhusein A, Bernstein CN (2012) 5-aminosalicylic acid is not protective against colorectal cancer in inflammatory bowel disease: a meta-analysis of non-referral populations. Am J Gastroenterol 107:1298–1304
97. van Schaik FD, van Oijen MG, Smeets HM et al (2012) Thiopurines prevent advanced colorectal neoplasia in patients with inflammatory bowel disease. Gut 61:235–240
98. Pasternak B, Svanström H, Schmiegelow K et al (2013) Use of azathioprine and the risk of cancer in inflammatory bowel disease. Am J Epidemiol 177:1296–1305
99. Armstrong RG, West J, Card TR (2010) Risk of cancer in inflammatory bowel disease treated with azathioprine: a UK population- based case-control study. Am J Gastroenterol 105:1604–1609
100. Onizawa M, Nagaishi T, Kanai T et al (2009) Signaling pathway via TNF-alpha/NF-kappaB in intestinal epithelial cells may be directly involved in colitis-associated carcinogenesis. Am J Physiol Gastrointest Liver Physiol 296:G850–G859
101. Andersen NN et al (2014) Association between tumor necrosis factor-α antagonists and risk of cancer in patients with inflammatory bowel disease. JAMA 311(23):2406–2413
102. Castaño-Milla C, Chaparro M, Gisbert JP (2014) Systematic review with meta-analysis: the declining risk of colorectal cancer in ulcerative colitis. Aliment Pharmacol Ther 39:645–659
103. Basu A, Wexner SD (2002) Perianal Crohn's disease. Curr Treat Opt Gastroenterol 5:197–206
104. Williamson PR, Hellinger MD, Larach SW et al (1995) A: Twenty-year review of the surgical management of perianal Crohn's disease. Dis Colon Rectum 38:389–392
105. Bernell O, Lapidus A, Hellers G (2001) Recurrence after colectomy in Crohn's colitis. Dis Colon Rectum 44:647–654
106. Lock MR, Fazio VW, Farmer RG et al (1981) Proximal recurrence and the fate of the rectum following excisional surgery for Crohn's disease of the large bowel. Ann Surg 194:754–760
107. Stern HS, Goldberg SM, Rothenberger DA et al (1984) Segmental versus total colectomy for large bowel Crohn's disease. World J Surg 8:118–122
108. Guillem JG, Roberts PL, Murray JJ et al (1992) Factors predictive of persistent or recurrent Crohn's disease in excluded rectal segments. Dis Colon Rectum 35:768–772
109. Yamamoto T, Bain IM, Allan RN et al (1999) Persistent perineal sinus after proctocolectomy for Crohn's disease. Dis Colon Rectum 42:96–101
110. Maeda Y, Heyckendorff-Diebold T, Tei TM et al (2011) Gracilis muscle transposition for complex fistula and persistent nonhealing sinus in perianal Crohn's disease. Inflamm Bowel Dis 17:583–589

Part II
Diagnosis

Chapter 4
Cancer Surveillance of Patients with Long-Standing Inflammatory Bowel Disease

Yoshiki Okita, Toshimitsu Araki, Koji Tanaka, Yuji Toiyama, Keiichi Uchida, and Masato Kusunoki

Abstract In response to the recognition of the higher risk of cancer in patients with inflammatory bowel disease (IBD), surveillance for those with long-standing disease has become an important tool in detecting and treating neoplastic lesions at an early stage and thus in the reduction of colitis-associated mortality. Most of the recent guidelines agree on the following: (1) For patients with proctosigmoiditis, a regular screening or surveillance colonoscopy program for detecting CRC is not necessary. (2) Surveillance colonoscopy should be started 6–10 years after the onset of symptoms for patients with left-sided or extensive colitis. (3) Ongoing surveillance colonoscopy should be carried out based on the individual risk profile. (4) Two to four random biopsy specimens should be taken every 10 cm along the entire colon, with additional samples acquired in suspicious areas. The random biopsy is now increasingly criticized because of its low yield in detecting neoplasia. In several guidelines, chromoendoscopy with targeted biopsies is an acceptable alternative to white light endoscopy with random biopsy. The value of other newer endoscopic techniques such as narrowband imaging, autofluorescence imaging, and fluorescence endoscopy, with targeted biopsies, remains to be determined.

Keywords Surveillance • Random biopsy • Targeted biopsy • Chromoendoscopy

4.1 Introduction

Crohn first described colorectal cancer (CRC) in association with inflammatory bowel disease (IBD) in 1925 [1]. Since then, the association between ulcerative colitis (UC) and carcinoma of the colon has been confirmed in numerous studies [2–5]. However, concerns remain regarding the adequate surveillance, diagnosis, and treatment of early preneoplastic and neoplastic lesions [6].

Y. Okita (✉) • T. Araki • K. Tanaka • Y. Toiyama • K. Uchida • M. Kusunoki
Department of Gastrointestinal and Pediatric Surgery, Mie University Graduate School of Medicine, 2-174 Edobashi, Tsu, Mie 514-8507, Japan
e-mail: nyokkin@clin.medic.mie-u.ac.jp

M. Kusunoki (ed.), *Colitis-Associated Cancer*, DOI 10.1007/978-4-431-55522-3_4

UC is a well-characterized chronic idiopathic form of IBD. The long-standing nature of UC and its relapsing and remitting course carry an increased risk for the development of colorectal neoplasia [7]. The overall prevalence of CRC in any UC patient was estimated to be 3.7 % in a large meta-analysis reported by Eaden et al. in 2001 [8]. Patients with a course of disease longer than 10 years and those with pancolitis are at the highest risk. Compared with the general population, patients with left-sided UC or those with more proximal disease are considered to be at greater risk for cancer development [9, 10].

Recent data have shown that colitis of Crohn's disease (CD) carries a similar magnitude of risk for the same disease extent. Canavan et al. [11] reported that the cumulative risk for patients with CD was 2.9 % at 10 years, 5.6 % at 20 years, and 8.3 % at 30 years after CD diagnosis and that, following a diagnosis of CD, the cumulative risk of developing CRC is comparable to the risk associated with UC [11].

Given the higher risk for cancer development, surveillance in patients with long-standing IBD has become an important tool in detecting and treating neoplastic lesions at an early stage and thus in the reduction of colitis-associated mortality [12]. Various guidelines, such as those of the European Crohn's and Colitis Organisation (ECCO), British Society of Gastroenterology (BSG), and American Gastroenterological Association (AGA), have been introduced to improve the detection of dysplasia and the management of surgically curable cancer and thereby the prognosis of these patients. This chapter provides a review of the current status of neoplasia surveillance in patients with long-standing IBD.

4.2 Risk Factors for Colitis-Associated Cancer in UC (Table 4.1)

Based on the long-term follow-up reported in a subset of the studies included in the meta-analysis by Eaden et al. [8], the cumulative risk of CRC in patients with left-sided disease or pancolitis was 1.6 % at 10 years, 8.3 % at 20 years, and 18.4 % at 30 years after the development of UC [8]. Several studies have shown a general consensus regarding little or no increased risk of CRC in patients with proctitis or proctosigmoiditis, an intermediate risk in those with left-sided colitis, and the highest risk in those with pancolitis. The meta-analysis by Eaden et al. [8] also reported an overall prevalence of 3.7 % for CRC among patients with UC in all 116 studies; however, when the analysis was restricted to the 35 studies that stratified their own analyses by extent of UC, the prevalence of CRC among patients with extensive involvement rose to 5.4 % [8, 13]. Disease duration and anatomic extent are well-established risk factors for the development of CRC.

Determination of anatomic extent in assessing cancer risk has historically been based on macroscopic rather than histologic inflammation. Both macroscopic and microscopic healing may occur, but once extensive colitis is documented, an

Table 4.1 Risk factor for colitis-associated cancer for ulcerative colitis

Extensive colitis
Primary sclerosing cholangitis
Severe long-standing inflammation
Inflammatory polyps
Colonic stricture
Family history of colorectal cancer, especially aged <50
Personal history of dysplasia

increased risk of cancer should be assumed depending on the greatest previously determined extent. Mathy et al. [14] reported that colitis-associated cancer in patients with UC may arise in endoscopically normal but histologically involved areas of the colon. They concluded that further studies are needed to determine the risk of colitis-related neoplasia in patients with microscopic pancolitis but limited gross disease.

A study from the Netherlands suggested that cancers will be missed if surveillance is commenced at 8–10 years for patients with pancolitis and at 15–20 years for patients with left-sided disease because 9–15 % of the cancers that developed in their study patients occurred before these time frames [15]. Indeed, up to 22 % of patients who develop a colitis-associated colon carcinoma do so prior to commencing surveillance colonoscopies. However, the majority of studies have shown that the incidence is very low at 10 years of disease, and might even be decreasing [8, 16–18].

The wide variation of risk estimates reported in the literature may be attributed to differences in additional risk factors in the patient cohorts studied. The most consistent risk factor reported is primary sclerosing cholangitis (PSC), which corresponds to a CRC risk up to 31 % [19–21]. Soetikno et al. [22] conducted a meta-analysis of 11 studies and found that, overall, 21 % of the patients with both UC and PSC developed colorectal neoplasms, compared with 4 % of the patients without PSC.

Histologic or clinical disease activity is regarded as a risk factor for colitis-associated cancer [7, 23, 24]. Postinflammatory polyps may be markers of previous inflammatory severity and are closely related to the neoplasm [7, 25, 26]. A case-control study of patients with UC from St. Mark's Hospital demonstrated that inflammatory polyps and colonic strictures increased the risk of CRC by twofold and fourfold, respectively, compared with individuals without these abnormalities [27]. In addition, a population-based cohort study reported that a family history of CRC was associated with a more than twofold higher risk of IBD-associated CRC [adjusted relative risk (RR) = 2.5; 95 % confidence interval (CI), 1.4–4.4]; furthermore, patients with a first-degree relative diagnosed with CRC before 50 years of age also had a higher risk (RR = 9.2; 95 % CI, 3.7–23) [28]. According to these data, the surveillance strategy for a particular patient should be determined based not only on the duration and extent of colitis but also on the presence of other risk factors.

4.3 Incidence and Prevalence of CD-Associated Cancer

Because of the chronic intestinal inflammation characteristic of the disease, CD is regarded as a risk factor for intestinal carcinoma. However, while some studies have reported that CD patients have an increased risk of cancer [29–35], other studies did not find any correlation [36–39]. In their 1994 study of the CRC risk in CD in a cohort of 281 patients, Gillen et al. [32] showed that those with extensive CD-associated colitis had an 18-fold higher risk, which decreased with increasing age at onset but increased significantly with a young age at onset.

A Canadian cohort study matched a population-based IBD database to a cancer registry in North America between 1984 and 1997 [34]. The incidence of CRC was higher in those with Crohn's colitis (RR = 2.64; 95 % CI, 1.69–4.12) or UC (RR = 2.75; 95 % CI, 1.91–3.97) than in the general population. That study also found a higher risk of rectal cancer in patients with UC (RR = 1.90; 95 % CI, 1.05–3.43) but not in those with Crohn's colitis (RR = 1.08; 95 % CI, 0.43–2.70).

Previous studies reported an increased risk of cancer in patients with CD of longer duration and extent [40, 41]. Stahl et al. [40] showed that patients with an early onset of CD were at higher risk for developing cancer; according to Maykel et al. [41], advanced age at CD diagnosis increased the risk of developing cancer [40, 41].

In the meta-analysis by von Roon et al. [42], based on 34 studies comprising 60,122 patients with CD, the RR of small bowel cancer or CRC compared with the baseline population was 28.4 (95 % CI, 14.46–55.66) and 2.4 (95 % CI, 1.56–4.36), respectively. In a subgroup analysis, patients with CD had an increased risk of colon cancer (RR = 2.59; 95 % CI, 1.54–4.36) but not of rectal cancer (RR = 1.46; 95 % CI, 0.8–2.55) [42].

The meta-analysis of Laukoetter et al. [43] consisted of 20 clinical studies with a total of 40,547 patients. The incidence of CD-associated cancer in CD patients was 0.8/1,000 person-years, meaning that during a 1-year observation period, 0.8 CD patients out of 1,000 developed CD-associated cancer. CD-associated CRC had a pooled incidence of 0.5/1,000 person-years (95 % CI, 0.3/1,000–0.6/1,000 person-years). The prevalence was 0.24 % (95 % CI, 0.19–0.28). The incidence of CRC and small bowel carcinoma in CD was 0.5/1,000 and 0.5/1,000 person-years, respectively. The pooled incidence of carcinomas in patients with fistulas was 0.2/1,000 person-years (95 % CI, 0.0/1,000–0.4/1,000 person-years). The mean duration between CD diagnosis and CD-associated cancer was 18.3 years. The authors concluded that although the risk of CRC is significantly increased in patients with CD, it is far lower than in those with long-standing UC. However, this meta-analysis did not find a significant relationship between cancer development and either the anatomic segments involved by CD or longer disease duration, although in the latter there was a trend toward a higher incidence. A stratification of cancer risk by disease duration has not been possible because of the paucity of appropriate studies [11].

Moreover, the benefit of surveillance colonoscopy in CD has yet to be established, and the early detection of small bowel carcinoma in patients with CD remains problematic. Routine magnetic resonance enteroclysis/enterography or capsule endoscopy could potentially detect these malignancies at an early stage, but the use of these methods to screen asymptomatic individuals is costly and has not been shown to prolong survival in patients with CD.

4.4 Timing of Initial Screening Colonoscopy and Surveillance Interval in Patients with UC (Table 4.2)

Most of the recent guidelines agree on the following: (1) For patients with proctosigmoiditis, regular screening or surveillance colonoscopy for detecting CRC is not necessary. (2) Surveillance colonoscopy should be started 6–10 years after the onset of symptoms for patients with left-sided or extensive colitis. (3) Ongoing surveillance colonoscopy should be carried out based on the individual risk profile.

There are some minor variations among the guidelines with respect to the timing of initial screening colonoscopy and the surveillance interval. In the guidelines of both the ECCO and the BSG, initial screening and surveillance colonoscopy for detecting CRC are determined based on risk stratification. The 2013 guideline of the ECCO recommends that patients with extensive UC as well as those with left-sided UC who have at least 8 years of disease beginning from the onset of symptoms should undergo screening colonoscopy. The ECCO's recommendations for surveillance colonoscopy are cited below [44]:

1. In all patients with UC irrespective of the disease activity, a screening colonoscopy could be carried out 6–8 years after the beginning of symptoms to assess the patient's individual risk profile.
2. When disease activity is limited to the rectum without evidence of previous or current endoscopic and/or microscopic inflammation proximal to the rectum, inclusion in a regular surveillance colonoscopy program is not necessary.
3. In cases with concurrent primary sclerosing cholangitis (PSC), surveillance colonoscopies should be carried out yearly from the point of PSC diagnosis irrespective of disease activity and extent.
4. The CRC risk profile should be determined at the screening colonoscopy or the first surveillance colonoscopy 6–8 years after the first manifestation. Risk stratification mainly depends on extent of disease, severity endoscopic and/or histological inflammation, pseudopolyps, concurrence of PSC, and family history of CRC.
5. The individual risk profile dictates surveillance colonoscopy intervals: every 1–2 years (high risk) or every 3–4 years (low risk) from the eighth year after the first manifestation in both extensive UC and left-sided UC.

Table 4.2 Comparison of screening recommendation from international guidelines for patients with colitis

	ECCO 2013	BSG 2010	AGA 2010	ACG 2010
First screening	6–8years	10 years	Maximum 8 years	8–10 years
Surveillance interval	High risk, 1–2 years	High risk, 1 year	1–3 years	8–10 years
	Low risk, every 3–4 years	Intermediate risk, 3 years	More often at high risk E.g., PSC	1–2 years
		Low risk, every 5 years		
Biopsy	Targeted biopsy with chromoendoscopy by trained endoscopist	Targeted biopsy with chromoendoscopy is recommended.	Random biopsy ($\geq$33) from each anatomic section	Multiple biopsies at regular intervals
	Quadrant biopsies every 10 cm	Two to four biopsies every 10 cm if no chromoendoscopy	Targeted biopsy with chromoendoscopy by trained endoscopist	Targeted biopsy with chromoendoscopy by trained endoscopist

ECCO European Crohn's and Colitis Organisation; *BSG* British Society of Gastroenterology; *AGA* American Gastroenterological Association; *ACG* American College of Gastroenterology; *PSC* primary sclerosing cholangitis

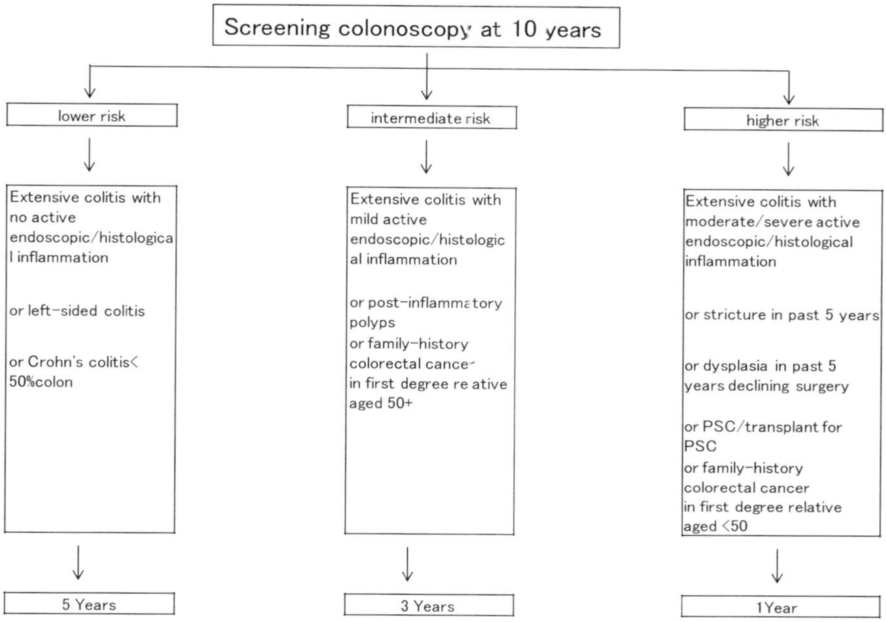

Fig. 4.1 Surveillance recommendations for patients with colitis from the British Society of Gastroenterology

In the BSG guideline, the surveillance colonoscopy program is decided upon based on the individual risk profile (Fig. 4.1). Screening colonoscopy and surveillance colonoscopy are recommended as follows [45]:

1. All patients with UC or Crohn's colitis should undergo a screening colonoscopy approximately 10 years after the onset of colitis symptoms to assess disease extent and other endoscopic risk factors.
2. Surveillance colonoscopies should be performed, where possible, when the disease is in remission. Surveillance procedure should not be unduly delayed if remission cannot be achieved.
3. The risk of cancer is influenced by the duration and extent of disease and additional risk factors (such as PSC and family history of CRC) and is also linked to the endoscopic and histologic appearances at colonoscopy.
4. If a dysplastic polyp is detected within an area of inflammation and can be removed in its entirety, it is not necessary to recommend colectomy.

According to the BSG, surveillance intervals are determined according to risk category (higher risk, yearly; moderate risk, every 3 years; higher risk, every 5 years).

The 2010 guideline of the AGA recommends that all patients, regardless of the extent of disease at initial diagnosis, undergo a screening colonoscopy at a maximum of 8 years after the onset of symptoms [46]. The AGA's recommendations for screening colonoscopy and surveillance colonoscopy are as follows:

1. All patients, regardless of the extent of disease at initial diagnosis, should undergo a screening colonoscopy a maximum of 8 years after onset of symptoms, with multiple biopsy specimens obtained throughout the entire colon, to assess the true microscopic extent of inflammation.
2. Patients with ulcerative proctitis or ulcerative proctosigmoiditis are not considered at increased risk for IBD-related CRC and thus may be managed on the basis of average-risk recommendations.
3. Patients with extensive or left-sided colitis, with a negative screening colonoscopy, should begin regular surveillance colonoscopy within 1–2 years.
4. After two negative examinations (no dysplasia or cancer), further surveillance examinations should be performed every 1–3 years. Increasing the frequency of surveillance colonoscopy to every 1–2 years after 20 years of disease is not needed for all patients but should be individualized according to the presence or absence of other risk factors.
5. Patients with PSC should begin surveillance colonoscopy at the time of this diagnosis and then undergo yearly colonoscopy thereafter.
6. Patients with a history of CRC in first-degree relatives, ongoing active endoscopic or histologic inflammation, or anatomic abnormalities such as a foreshortened colon, stricture, or multiple inflammatory pseudopolyps may benefit from more frequent surveillance examinations.

The 2010 American College of Gastroenterology guideline recommends that initial screening should be started after 8–10 years of colitis in patients with either left-sided colitis or pancolitis and annual or biannual surveillance should be performed [47].

The 2006 guideline for the management of UC in Japan recommends that surveillance colonoscopy should be started 8–10 years after disease onset for patients with extensive colitis and annual or biannual colonoscopy, including biopsies, beginning 8–10 years after disease onset in patients with extensive colitis [48]. In this guideline, surveillance colonoscopy for detecting CRC is not determined based on risk stratification.

4.5 Sampling Method: Step Biopsy or Target Biopsy? (Table 4.2)

While surveillance colonoscopy allows the early detection and treatment of CRC, especially in patients with long-standing UC, the flat or diffuse infiltrative macroscopic lesions that sometimes arise in UC are difficult to see endoscopically. In their 1986 study, Broström et al. [49] examined the use of surveillance colonoscopy for the early detection of dysplasia. The entire colon was separated into ten segments, and two biopsies were taken at each one. Manning et al. [50] reported the results of a prospective study of screening for colorectal epithelial dysplasia by regular colonoscopy. In their 1987 study, biopsy specimens were taken from flat mucosa at approximately 8–10-cm intervals along the colon and rectum and from any identifiable mass lesions. Based on these and other studies of surveillance colonoscopy, the practice of multiple biopsies in patients with long-standing UC during surveillance colonoscopy has been widely adopted.

Rubin et al. [51] used a mathematical model to show that 33 biopsy specimens were needed to detect dysplasia with 90 % probability, if dysplasia is present. At least 64 biopsy specimens were needed to reach a 95 % probability of detecting dysplasia. That study provided the basis for surveillance practice recommendations. Current guidelines for dysplasia surveillance recommend quadrant-based random biopsies every 10 cm throughout the entire colon and a minimum of 33 biopsies [44–47]. However, random biopsy samples only 0.03 % of the mucosal surface, has a detection rate of <2 per 1,000 biopsies [52], and does not affect clinical decision-making when advanced techniques are used [53]. Broek et al. [52] retrospectively analyzed 466 surveillance colonoscopies (in 167 patients) during which 11,772 random biopsies were obtained. The authors concluded that the low yield and lack of clinical consequences from random biopsies question its necessity and cost-effectiveness in UC surveillance. Thus, chromoendoscopy (CE) provides an alternative to colonoscopy with random biopsies, and its use is supported in recent guidelines [44, 45].

Moreover, recent data have shown that most gastroenterologists do not follow the recommended biopsy protocol. In a study from the Netherlands, only 27 % of gastroenterologists complied with the recommended number of 33 random biopsies [54]. Eaden et al. [55, 56] used a questionnaire to show that >50 % of the gastroenterologists surveyed obtained fewer than ten colonic mucosal biopsies per endoscopic surveillance examination.

The BSG guideline recommends pancolonic dye spraying with the targeted biopsy of abnormal areas; otherwise, two to four random biopsy specimens from every 10 cm of the colorectum should be taken, with additional biopsies of suspicious areas.

The Research Group of Intractable Inflammatory Bowel Disease of the Ministry of Health, Labour and Welfare of Japan is carrying out a randomized controlled study to compare the efficacy of step biopsy and target biopsy [57]. The results of this study will soon be available.

4.6 Chromoendoscopy and Other Newer Endoscopic Techniques

4.6.1 Chromoendoscopy

Target biopsy techniques have gained increasing acceptance [58]. Among these newer techniques CE is the most well established, and it has been used to better define the superficial gastrointestinal mucosa [59]. CE involves the topical application of a dye onto the colonic mucosa. It has two main advantages [27]: (1) it improves the detection of subtle colonic lesions, which raises the sensitivity of the endoscopic examination, and (2) once a lesion is detected, its CE appearance can aid in its characterization, which raises the specificity of the endoscopic examination [46, 56]. Previous studies demonstrated that the use of CE increases the detection rate of dysplasia by two- to threefold, corresponding to a per lesion increase of four- to fivefold [60–62].

Use of a magnifying colonoscope may further increase the sensitivity and specificity of CE [46]. Crypt architecture can be categorized by evaluating the pit pattern, which aides in the differentiation between neoplastic and nonneoplastic changes and in the performance of targeted biopsies [63].

The different stains used in CE can be classified as absorptive or contrast agents [59]. Absorptive agents include methylene blue (0.1–0.5 %) and cresyl violet (0.2 %). They are rapidly absorbed by normal colonic mucosa but poorly absorbed by dysplastic or inflamed tissue, thus enhancing the superficial structure of lesions and demonstrating the various cell types. Contrast agents, such as indigo carmine, pool in the mucosal grooves without reaction and absorption and thus highlight the superficial structure of lesions.

Several studies have evaluated the use of CE as an adjunctive method to diagnose dysplasia or cancer, based on its ability to more accurately evaluate the extent of disease and the degree of inflammatory activity [60, 62, 64–66]. In the study of Kiesslich et al. [64], patients with long-standing UC were assigned to conventional colonoscopy or colonoscopy with CE using methylene blue. The correlation between the endoscopic assessment of both the degree and the extent of colonic inflammation was better in the CE group than in patients examined with conventional colonoscopy. In addition, more targeted biopsies were possible with CE, and significantly more dysplasia was detected. The sensitivity and specificity for the differentiation of nonneoplastic from neoplastic lesions were both 93 %.

In a randomized control study, Rutter et al. [60] evaluated 100 patients with long-standing extensive UC who underwent "back to back" colonoscopies with both random and targeted biopsies, followed by spraying with indigo carmine and biopsies. Median extubation times for the first and second colonoscopies were 11 and 10 min, respectively. During conventional colonoscopy, 43 mucosal abnormalities were detected, of which two were dysplastic. Following dye spraying, 114 additional abnormalities were detected, of which seven were dysplastic. The targeted biopsy protocol detected dysplasia in significantly more patients than achieved with the nontargeted protocol [60].

Hurlstone et al. [66] analyzed 350 patients with long-standing UC who underwent surveillance colonoscopy using high-magnification CE. Quadrant-based biopsies at 10-cm intervals were taken on extubation, in addition to targeted biopsies of abnormal mucosal areas. The data were compared to those from 350 control patients, matched for disease duration and extent, who had undergone conventional colonoscopic surveillance. Significantly more intraepithelial neoplastic lesions were detected in the magnification chromoscopy group than in the controls (69 vs. 24 lesions, $P < 0.0001$). In addition, a greater number of flat lesions with intraepithelial neoplasia were detected in the CE group than in controls (53 vs. 14 lesions, $P < 0.001$). The authors concluded that magnification CE can predict neoplastic and nonneoplastic mucosal changes with a high overall accuracy [66].

4.6.2 Virtual Chromoendoscopy

Newer endoscopic techniques are being explored to aid in the diagnosis of dysplasia in IBD, although none has yet been rigorously studied. These new techniques include virtual chromoendoscopy (VCE), narrow band imaging (NBI) [67], fluorescence endoscopy [68, 69], optical coherence tomography [70], and confocal endomicroscopy [61, 70, 71].

VCE, also called dye-less chromoendoscopy, is a recently developed imaging technique that comprises NBI (Olympus, Tokyo, Japan), Fujinon intelligent color enhancement (FICE; Fujinon, Tokyo, Japan), and i-Scan (Pentax, Tokyo, Japan). NBI provides clear imaging of the microvascular structure of the colon. Its development was motivated by the quest for a simpler technique that would obviate the complexity of CE [67]. This unique form of electronic CE was first described by Gono et al. [72]. The method is based on illumination of the mucosal surface by light with a defined narrow band of wavelengths. Two narrow bands, centered at 415 (blue light) and 540 nm (green light), are used in the system introduced by Olympus (Olympus Medical, Tokyo, Japan). These selected wavelengths can pass through the mucosa to a defined depth, and their absorption correlates with the absorption maximum of a molecule of hemoglobin. A wavelength of 415 nm penetrates only the very superficial layers of the mucosa and is absorbed by blood in the intrapapillary capillary loops. The narrow band centered at 540 nm penetrates the deeper level and accentuates the venules and arterioles located under a layer of intrapapillary capillary loops. Using NBI to illuminate the mucosal membrane substantially increases the contrast between blood-containing vessels and the surrounding tissues, allowing even very subtle changes in the microvascular architecture to be identified [73].

Dekker et al. [67] carried out a prospective, randomized, crossover study of 42 patients with long-standing UC and compared the accuracy of NBI with that of standard colonoscopy for the detection of neoplasia. Using NBI, 52 visible lesions were identified in 17 patients, whereas with standard WLE, 28 lesions were detected in 13 patients. Pathologic evaluation of targeted biopsies identified 11 patients with neoplasia. Neoplasia was detected by both techniques in four patients but only by NBI or conventional colonoscopy in four and three patients, respectively. The sensitivity of that first-generation NBI system for the detection of neoplasia was comparable to that of conventional colonoscopy, although a larger number of suspicious lesions were found during NBI. The authors concluded that it is still too early to stop taking additional random biopsies at surveillance colonoscopy in patients with UC [67].

Two other trials demonstrated that high-definition WLE was equivalent to NBI [74, 75]. In the study of van den Broek et al. [74], 11 out of 16 (69 %) neoplastic lesions were detected by high-definition WLE and 13 out of 16 by NBI (81 %) ($P = 0.727$). In the study of Ignjatovic et al. [75], there was no difference in the proportion of patients with at least one area of dysplasia detected by WLE vs. by NBI, with five patients having at least one dysplastic lesion in each group [odds ratio (OR) = 1.00; 95 % CI, 0.27–3.67; $P = 1.00$]. This remained unchanged when adjusted for other variables (OR = 0.69; 95 % CI, 0.16–2.96; $P = 0.62$).

Efthymiou et al. [76] evaluated 44 patients with IBD to compare CE and NBI with respect to lesion detection and to assess the accuracy of the mucosal pit pattern (Kudo classification) as seen on NBI in predicting mucosal histology. CE identified more lesions than NBI (131 vs. 102, $P < 0.001$), detecting 23 neoplastic (dysplastic or indefinite for dysplasia) lesions in 11 patients compared with the 20 lesions in 10 patients detected by NBI ($P = 0.180$). Kudo classification by NBI had a low sensitivity and modest accuracy for dysplasia (42 % and 74 %, respectively). The authors concluded that there was a nonsignificant trend in favor of CE for the detection of dysplasia and that NBI cannot be recommended as an alternative to CE for dysplasia surveillance [76].

Pellisé et al. [77] examined the number of false-positive and true-positive lesions in patients undergoing CE and NBI as well as the proportion of patients with missed intraepithelial neoplasia lesions. In the per-lesion analysis, NBI had a significantly lower false-positive biopsy rate ($P = 0.001$) and a similar true-positive rate [77]. The efficacy of NBI in the endoscopy-based differential diagnosis of sporadic neoplasia vs. colitis-associated dysplasia or cancer remains to be confirmed [78].

4.6.3 Autofluorescence Imaging

Autofluorescence imaging (AFI) is a novel technique that takes advantage of the fluorescence of tissues exposed to ultraviolet (<400 nm) or short-wavelength visible (mostly blue) light. The autofluorescence produced by certain molecules (fluorophores) has a longer wavelength than that of the excitation light [59, 79]. Tissue autofluorescence is influenced by several factors, including the architecture and light absorption properties of the tissues (the latter is mainly determined by the concentration of hemoglobin in the tissues), their biochemical environment, and their metabolic status [59, 80]. These features are distinct in neoplasia, as the greenish background of normal colonic tissue is replaced by a purple-colored mucosa [59].

In their prospective pilot trial ($n = 50$) using a randomized crossover design between standard targeted WLE biopsies and AFI-targeted biopsies, van den Broek et al. [81] demonstrated significantly better detection in the AFI-first group, in which ten neoplastic lesions were detected among 25 patients, while WLE did not detect any additional lesions. In the WLE-first group, three lesions were detected among 25 patients, and subsequent AFI detected three more ($P = 0.036$). This study reported that the Kudo classification by NBI had a sensitivity and specificity of 75 % and 81 %, respectively, but on AFI all neoplasias were purple (sensitivity 100 %) [81].

A comparison of the effectiveness of AFI vs. CE in IBD has yet to be published.

4.6.4 *Fluorescence Endoscopy*

Sensitizers are molecules that accumulate selectively in malignant and premalignant tissue and fluoresce under blue light excitation; thus, they are highly useful in targeted biopsies. 5-Aminolevulinic acid (5-ALA), a prodrug in heme biosynthesis, is converted intracellularly into the sensitizing agent protoporphyrin IX. Due to the low ferrochelatase activity of tumor cells, protoporphyrin IX accumulates selectively in neoplastic tissue [82] and thus allows the detection of dysplasia by typical red fluorescence after illumination with blue light. Promising results for fluorescence endoscopy of bronchial [83] and bladder [84] tumors after 5-ALA sensitization have been reported.

Messmann et al. [69] assessed the efficacy of fluorescence endoscopy after 5-ALA sensitization for detecting dysplasia in UC. Optically guided biopsies were performed with fluorescence endoscopy after oral (20 mg/kg) or local (either with an enema or by spraying the mucosa via a catheter) sensitization with 5-ALA. In their study, the sensitivity of fluorescence endoscopy for dysplastic lesions was 87–100 % after local sensitization. The authors concluded that fluorescence endoscopy after 5-ALA sensitization can be used to visualize dysplastic lesions [69].

4.6.5 *Confocal Laser Endomicroscopy*

Confocal laser endomicroscopy is a promising method that allows for instant in vivo histology during ongoing endoscopy, but limited data regarding its use are available [56].

Two probe devices have been approved: one is integrated into the distal tip of a high-resolution endoscope (iCLE; Pentax, Tokyo, Japan), and the other is a stand-alone probe that is introduced through the instrument channel of standard endoscopes (pCLE; Cellvizio, Mauna Kea Technologies, Paris, France) [59, 71]. The functional principle is based on the fluorescence of mucosal tissue when exposed to blue laser light at an excitation wavelength of 488 nm, with light emission detected at 505 nm [59]. The resulting images provide an approximately 1,000-fold magnification of the tissue in vivo [71]. For confocal imaging, a fluorescence agent is administered either systemically (fluorescein sodium) or topically (e.g., acriflavine or cresyl violet) with fluorescein sodium [85]. Kiesslich et al. [61] conducted a randomized controlled trial to assess the effectiveness of combined CE and endomicroscopy in the diagnosis of intraepithelial neoplasias. They randomized

161 patients with UC in remission either to conventional colonoscopy or to chromoscopy with endomicroscopy to detect dysplasia or CRC. In the conventional colonoscopy group ($n = 73$), random and targeted biopsy examinations were performed. In the endomicroscopy group ($n = 80$), circumscribed mucosal lesions were identified by chromoscopy and evaluated for targeted biopsy by endomicroscopy. By using chromoscopy with endomicroscopy, the number of neoplasias that could be detected increased by 4.75-fold ($P = 0.005$) compared with conventional colonoscopy, but 50 % fewer biopsy specimens ($P = 0.008$) were required. The presence of neoplastic changes was predicted with high accuracy (94.7 % sensitivity, 98.3 % specificity, and 97.8 % accuracy). The authors concluded that endomicroscopy based on in vivo histology can determine whether UC lesions identified by chromoscopy should undergo biopsy examination, thereby increasing the diagnostic yield and reducing the need for biopsy examinations [61].

Hurlstone et al. [86] performed a prospective randomized controlled study to compare the diagnostic yield of intraepithelial neoplasia and cancer in patients undergoing UC screening using chromoscopy-assisted endomicroscopy vs. pancolonic chromoscopy-assisted colonoscopy. Endomicroscopy-targeted biopsies increased the diagnostic yield of intraepithelial neoplasia compared to chromoscopy-guided biopsies alone by 2.5-fold [86]. In addition to the improved detection, chromoscopy-guided endomicroscopy offers considerable cost savings.

4.7 Effectiveness of Cancer Surveillance in Reducing CRC-Related Death in UC

As noted above (Sect. 4.5), UC-associated CRC sometimes occurs as flat or diffuse infiltrative macroscopic lesions that are difficult to see endoscopically. Dysplasia is considered to be a precancerous lesion, and its presence is associated with a high likelihood of a complicating cancer, either nearby or in another region. Therefore, in surveillance colonoscopy, dysplasia is considered as a useful marker for detecting UC-associated CRC [87–89]. Accordingly, any screening or surveillance program must include a search for dysplastic alterations, to enable their treatment and to prevent the development of invasive cancer. While prophylactic proctocolectomy eliminates the risk of CRC, this strategy is not acceptable to most patients or physicians [90]. However, no randomized controlled trials have been performed to verify that surveillance colonoscopy is effective. A previous Japanese study reported that close surveillance results in the detection of 48 % of the cancers, 61 % of which are early cancers [91].

In 2006, the Cochrane Database of Systematic Review assessed the effectiveness of cancer surveillance programs in reducing the death rate from CRC in patients with UC and colonic CD [92, 93]. Three case-control studies were examined. In a population-based, nested case-control study of 142 patients with UC (derived from a study population of 4,664 patients with UC) reported by Karlen et al. [94], two of the 40 patients with UC and CRC who died and 18 of the 102 matched controls with UC and CRC who were alive at the time of the death of the patient had undergone at least one surveillance colonoscopy (RR = 0.28; 95 % CI, 0.07–1.31) [94]. One of the 40 patients who died had undergone surveillance colonoscopies on two or more occasions compared with 12 out of the 102 controls (RR = 0.22; 95 % CI, 0.03–1.74).

In a study published in 1993, Choi et al. [95] examined 41 patients who developed CRC. Fifteen of the 19 patients had Dukes' A or B carcinoma in the surveillance group compared with nine out of 22 patients in the non-surveillance group ($P = 0.039$). The 5-year survival rate was 77.2 % in the surveillance group and 36.3 % in the non-surveillance group ($P = 0.026$). Four of the 19 patients in the surveillance group died from CRC compared to 11 of the 22 patients in the non-surveillance group (RR = 0.42; 95 % CI, 0.16–1.11).

In the 1991 study of Lashner et al. [96], four of 91 patients who underwent surveillance died of CRC, compared with two of 95 patients who did not undergo surveillance (RR = 2.09; 95 % CI, 0.39–11.12). Colectomy was less common in the surveillance group (33 vs. 51; $P < 0.05$) and was performed, on average, 4 years later (after 10 years of disease) than in the non-surveillance group, although improvement was not related to the anticipated benefits of improved cancer-related survival.

The review concluded that, for patients with UC undergoing surveillance, cancer tend to be detected at an earlier stage and patients therefore have a better prognosis, even if lead-time bias may contribute to the apparent benefit of surveillance. Indirect evidence supports the effectiveness of surveillance in reducing the risk of death from IBD-associated CRC and suggests that surveillance is cost-effective, although there is no clear evidence that it prolongs survival in patients with extensive colitis [92, 93].

4.8 Initial Screening and Surveillance Programs in Patients with CD

The effectiveness of surveillance in Crohn's colitis has been assessed in only a few studies. Friedman et al. [97] analyzed 1,424 examinations of 259 patients. On screening examination, definite dysplasia or cancer was found in 18 patients (7 %) (low-grade dysplasia, 13; high-grade dysplasia, 2; cancer, 3). On surveillance examinations, an additional 30 patients (14 %) had a first finding of definite dysplasia or cancer (low-grade dysplasia, 22; high-grade dysplasia, 4; cancer, 4). However, the appropriate screening and surveillance programs for long-standing CD have not been established yet.

The Crohn's & Colitis Foundation of America consensus conference recommendations for surveillance colonoscopy in patients with CD of the colon are as follows [98]:

1. Patients with major colonic involvement (at least one-third of the colon involved) who have harbored disease for 8–10 years from onset of symptoms should undergo a screening colonoscopy.
2. If no dysplasia or cancer is detected, a surveillance examination protocol should be started within 2 years.
3. After a negative surveillance colonoscopy, subsequent surveillance should be performed every 1–2 years. With two negative examinations, the next surveillance examination may be performed in 1–3 years until Crohn's colitis has been present for 20 years. At that time, surveillance should be performed every 1–2 years.

The BSG guideline recommends that all patients, not only those with UC but also those with Crohn's colitis, should undergo a screening colonoscopy approximately 10 years after the onset of colitis symptoms to assess disease extent and other endoscopic risk factors [45].

The AGA Institute Technical Review for surveillance colonoscopy in IBD recommends screening and surveillance not only for patients with long-standing UC but also for those with Crohn's colitis who have a disease involving at least one-third of the length of the colon [46].

There are currently no screening and surveillance programs aimed at detecting small bowel cancer. Further investigation, including a detailed meta-analysis of individual patients, is required to fully elucidate the risk of CRC and small bowel cancer in patients with CD [11].

4.9 Surveillance for Cancer Associated in CD Patients with Perianal Fistulas

Thomas et al. [99] analyzed 61 cases of cancer arising from perineal fistulas in patients with CD and found that a malignancy was suspected and proven in only 20 % of the patients on initial examination. Symptoms in patients with cancer arising from perineal fistulas in CD are usually nonspecific. A high level of attention must be paid to patients with long-standing perianal disease who have a change in symptoms. Clinical inspection or endoscopic examination is often insufficient because of anal pain and stricture, which may limit proper examination without anesthesia and in some cases even with anesthesia. Imaging studies including computed tomography, magnetic resonance imaging, or 18F-fluorodeoxyglucose positron emission tomography have a low sensitivity for detecting cancer in these patients [100,101]. Therefore, scheduled examinations and biopsy under anesthesia are necessary to diagnose anorectal cancer arising from a long-standing perianal fistula in CD [101].

A multicenter pilot study to determine an appropriate surveillance program for cancer arising from perineal fistulas in patients with CD is currently underway in

Japan, with Health and Labour Sciences Research Grants from the Ministry of Health, Labour and Welfare.

4.10 Factors Influencing the Success of Surveillance Colonoscopy

4.10.1 Precise Endoscopic Diagnosis

The endoscopic detection of dysplasia can be challenging and depends on the skills of the endoscopist. In a retrospective study, even after excluding polypoid cancers and apparent tubular adenomas, only approximately two-thirds of dysplastic lesions in patients with UC were visible [65]. Not all dysplastic lesions in IBD colons are visible with WLE, CE, and the newer high-definition colonoscopes. Surveillance colonoscopy should be performed on patients during clinical remission, to avoid confusing inflammatory changes with dysplasia [12]. Anatomic factors such as strictures and inflammatory pseudopolyps may interfere with the ability to detect or sample colonic dysplasia or cancer [46]. High-quality bowel cleansing and inactive mucosal disease are important to the success of a detailed mucosal examination [59].

4.10.2 Precise Histopathologic Diagnosis

Therapeutic recommendations for the management of dysplasia in UC are based on a macroscopic pattern (flat or elevated) and the microscopic characteristics of the lesion (indefinite, low-grade, or high-grade). Dysplasia almost certainly evolves along a progressive (continuous) scale rather than in discrete steps. Therefore, the interpretation of the grade of dysplasia varies even among experienced gastrointestinal pathologists [44, 102, 103]. Specimens with high-grade dysplasia are often considered negative, whereas those with indefinite and low-grade dysplasia are evaluated inconsistently. These limitations in the assessment of dysplasia have led to the recommendation that histologic findings should be confirmed by a second expert gastrointestinal pathologist [44].

4.10.3 Adequacy of Mucosal Sampling

The success of surveillance also depends on the adequacy of mucosal sampling. Detection of dysplasia may be affected by the number of biopsy specimens obtained at colonoscopy. Guidelines for surveillance colonoscopy in the United States and Europe recommend the use of step biopsy [46].

4.10.4 Frequency of Surveillance

The frequency of surveillance may influence the success of a surveillance program. The precise interval for performing surveillance colonoscopies has not been rigorously studied [46]. Indeed, dysplasia or cancer has been detected within 2 years of a negative surveillance colonoscopy [104, 105].

4.10.5 Patient Acceptance

Patient acceptance is important to the success of surveillance [104, 106]. In a case-control study by Eaden et al. of 102 cases of CRC in UC, more than two yearly visits to the hospital physician were associated with a decreased risk of developing CRC [107].

References

1. Crohn B (1925) The sigmoidoscopic picture of chronic ulcerative colitis (non-specific). Am J Med Sci 170:220–228
2. Bargen JA (1928) Chronic ulcerative colitis associated with malignant disease. Arch Surg 17:561–576
3. Bargen JA, Jackman RJ, Kerr JG (1938) Studies on the life histories of patients with chronic ulcerative colitis (thromboulcerative colitis) with some suggestions for treatment. Ann Intern Med 12:339–352
4. Sauer WGBJ (1944) Chronic ulcerative colitis followed by carcinoma: report of 26 cases. Proc Mayo Clin 19:311–315
5. Cattell RBBE (1947) The importance of malignant degeneration as a complication of chronic ulcerative colitis. Gastroenterology 8:695–710
6. Neumann H, Vieth M, Langner C et al (2011) Cancer risk in IBD: how to diagnose and how to manage DALM and ALM. World J Gastroenterol 17:3184–3191
7. Rutter M, Saunders B, Wilkinson K et al (2004) Severity of inflammation is a risk factor for colorectal neoplasia in ulcerative colitis. Gastroenterology 126:451–459
8. Eaden JA, Abrams KR, Mayberry JF (2001) The risk of colorectal cancer in ulcerative colitis: a meta-analysis. Gut 48:526–535
9. Ullman T, Odze R, Farraye FA (2009) Diagnosis and management of dysplasia in patients with ulcerative colitis and Crohn's disease of the colon. Inflamm Bowel Dis 15:630–638
10. Ekbom A, Helmick C, Zack M et al (1990) Ulcerative colitis and colorectal cancer. A population-based study. N Engl J Med 323:1228–1233
11. Canavan C, Abrams KR, Mayberry J (2006) Meta-analysis: colorectal and small bowel cancer risk in patients with Crohn's disease. Aliment Pharmacol Ther 23:1097–1104

12. Kim ER, Chang DK (2014) Colorectal cancer in inflammatory bowel disease: the risk, pathogenesis, prevention and diagnosis. World J Gastroenterol 20:9872–9881
13. Lakatos PL, Lakatos L (2008) Risk for colorectal cancer in ulcerative colitis: changes, causes and management strategies. World J Gastroenterol 14:3937–3947
14. Mathy C, Schneider K, Chen YY et al (2003) Gross versus microscopic pancolitis and the occurrence of neoplasia in ulcerative colitis. Inflamm Bowel Dis 9:351–355
15. Lutgens MW, Vleggaar FP, Schipper ME et al (2008) High frequency of early colorectal cancer in inflammatory bowel disease. Gut 57:1246–1251
16. Rutter MD, Saunders BP, Wilkinson KH et al (2006) Thirty-year analysis of a colonoscopic surveillance program for neoplasia in ulcerative colitis. Gastroenterology 130:1030–1038
17. Jess T, Loftus EV Jr, Velayos FS et al (2006) Risk of intestinal cancer in inflammatory bowel disease: a population-based study from olmsted county, Minnesota. Gastroenterology 130:1039–1046
18. Loftus EV Jr (2006) Epidemiology and risk factors for colorectal dysplasia and cancer in ulcerative colitis. Gastroenterol Clin North Am 35:517–531
19. Claessen MM, Vleggaar FP, Tytgat KM et al (2009) High lifetime risk of cancer in primary sclerosing cholangitis. J Hepatol 50:158–164
20. Bergeron V, Vienne A, Sokol H et al (2010) Risk factors for neoplasia in inflammatory bowel disease patients with pancolitis. Am J Gastroenterol 105:2405–2411
21. Jayaram H, Satsangi J, Chapman RW (2001) Increased colorectal neoplasia in chronic ulcerative colitis complicated by primary sclerosing cholangitis: fact or fiction? Gut 48:430–434
22. Soetikno RM, Lin OS, Heidenreich PA et al (2002) Increased risk of colorectal neoplasia in patients with primary sclerosing cholangitis and ulcerative colitis: a meta-analysis. Gastrointest Endosc 56:48–54
23. Gupta RB, Harpaz N, Itzkowitz S et al (2007) Histologic inflammation is a risk factor for progression to colorectal neoplasia in ulcerative colitis: a cohort study. Gastroenterology 133:1099–1105, quiz 1340–1091
24. Jess T, Loftus EV Jr, Velayos FS et al (2007) Risk factors for colorectal neoplasia in inflammatory bowel disease: a nested case-control study from Copenhagen county, Denmark and Olmsted county, Minnesota. Am J Gastroenterol 102:829–836
25. Baars JE, Looman CW, Steyerberg EW et al (2011) The risk of inflammatory bowel disease-related colorectal carcinoma is limited: results from a nationwide nested case-control study. Am J Gastroenterol 106:319–328
26. Velayos FS, Loftus EV Jr, Jess T et al (2006) Predictive and protective factors associated with colorectal cancer in ulcerative colitis: a case-control study. Gastroenterology 130:1941–1949
27. Rutter MD, Saunders BP, Wilkinson KH et al (2004) Cancer surveillance in longstanding ulcerative colitis: endoscopic appearances help predict cancer risk. Gut 53:1813–1816
28. Askling J, Dickman PW, Karlen P et al (2001) Family history as a risk factor for colorectal cancer in inflammatory bowel disease. Gastroenterology 120:1356–1362
29. Greenstein AJ, Sachar DB, Smith H et al (1981) A comparison of cancer risk in Crohn's disease and ulcerative colitis. Cancer 48:2742–2745
30. Munkholm P, Langholz E, Davidsen M et al (1993) Intestinal cancer risk and mortality in patients with Crohn's disease. Gastroenterology 105:1716–1723
31. Persson PG, Karlen P, Bernell O et al (1994) Crohn's disease and cancer: a population-based cohort study. Gastroenterology 107:1675–1679
32. Gillen CD, Andrews HA, Prior P et al (1994) Crohn's disease and colorectal cancer. Gut 35:651–655
33. Gillen CD, Walmsley RS, Prior P et al (1994) Ulcerative colitis and Crohn's disease: a comparison of the colorectal cancer risk in extensive colitis. Gut 35:1590–1592
34. Bernstein CN, Blanchard JF, Kliewer E et al (2001) Cancer risk in patients with inflammatory bowel disease: a population-based study. Cancer 91:854–862

35. Dossett LA, White LM, Welch DC et al (2007) Small bowel adenocarcinoma complicating Crohn's disease: case series and review of the literature. Am Surg 73:1181–1187
36. Gyde SN, Prior P, Macartney JC et al (1980) Malignancy in Crohn's disease. Gut 21:1024–1029
37. Weedon DD, Shorter RG, Ilstrup DM et al (1973) Crohn's disease and cancer. N Engl J Med 289:1099–1103
38. Gollop JH, Phillips SF, Melton LJ 3rd et al (1988) Epidemiologic aspects of Crohn's disease: a population based study in Olmsted County, Minnesota, 1943–1982. Gut 29:49–56
39. Ekbom A, Helmick C, Zack M et al (1991) The epidemiology of inflammatory bowel disease: a large, population-based study in Sweden. Gastroenterology 100:350–358
40. Stahl TJ, Schoetz DJ Jr, Roberts PL et al (1992) Crohn's disease and carcinoma: increasing justification for surveillance? Dis Colon Rectum 35:850–856
41. Maykel JA, Hagerman G, Mellgren AF et al (2006) Crohn's colitis: the incidence of dysplasia and adenocarcinoma in surgical patients. Dis Colon Rectum 49:950–957
42. von Roon AC, Reese G, Teare J et al (2007) The risk of cancer in patients with Crohn's disease. Dis Colon Rectum 50:839–855
43. Laukoetter MG, Mennigen R, Hannig CM et al (2011) Intestinal cancer risk in Crohn's disease: a meta-analysis. J Gastrointest Surg 15:576–583
44. Van Assche G, Dignass A, Bokemeyer B et al (2013) Second European evidence-based consensus on the diagnosis and management of ulcerative colitis part 3: special situations. J Crohns Colitis 7:1–33
45. Cairns SR, Scholefield JH, Steele RJ et al (2010) Guidelines for colorectal cancer screening and surveillance in moderate and high risk groups (update from 2002). Gut 59:666–689
46. Farraye FA, Odze RD, Eaden J et al (2010) AGA technical review on the diagnosis and management of colorectal neoplasia in inflammatory bowel disease. Gastroenterology 138:746–774, 774 e741–744; quiz e712–743
47. Kornbluth A, Sachar DB, Practice Parameters Committee of the American College of G (2010) Ulcerative colitis practice guidelines in adults: American College Of Gastroenterology, Practice Parameters Committee. Am J Gastroenterol 105:501–523, quiz 524
48. Matsuoka KT-CL (2010) Guidelines of the management of ulcerative colitis in Japan-Developed through integration of evidence and consensus among experts. IBD Res 4:189–239
49. Brostrom O, Lofberg R, Ost A et al (1986) Cancer surveillance of patients with longstanding ulcerative colitis: a clinical, endoscopical, and histological study. Gut 27:1408–1413
50. Manning AP, Bulgim OR, Dixon MF et al (1987) Screening by colonoscopy for colonic epithelial dysplasia in inflammatory bowel disease. Gut 28:1489–1494
51. Rubin CE, Haggitt RC, Burmer GC et al (1992) DNA aneuploidy in colonic biopsies predicts future development of dysplasia in ulcerative colitis. Gastroenterology 103:1611–1620
52. van den Broek FJ, Stokkers PC, Reitsma JB et al (2014) Random biopsies taken during colonoscopic surveillance of patients with longstanding ulcerative colitis: low yield and absence of clinical consequences. Am J Gastroenterol 109:715–722
53. East JE (2012) Colonoscopic cancer surveillance in inflammatory bowel disease: what's new beyond random biopsy? Clin Endosc 45:274–277
54. van Rijn AF, Fockens P, Siersema PD et al (2009) Adherence to surveillance guidelines for dysplasia and colorectal carcinoma in ulcerative and Crohn's colitis patients in the Netherlands. World J Gastroenterol 15:226–230
55. Eaden JA, Ward BA, Mayberry JF (2000) How gastroenterologists screen for colonic cancer in ulcerative colitis: an analysis of performance. Gastrointest Endosc 51:123–128
56. Guagnozzi D, Lucendo AJ (2012) Colorectal cancer surveillance in patients with inflammatory bowel disease: what is new? World J Gastrointest Endosc 4:108–116
57. Watanabe T, Ajioka Y, Matsumoto T et al (2011) Target biopsy or step biopsy? Optimal surveillance for ulcerative colitis: a Japanese nationwide randomized controlled trial. J Gastroenterol 46(Suppl 1):11–16

58. Tontini GE, Vecchi M, Neurath MF et al (2013) Review article: newer optical and digital chromoendoscopy techniques vs. dye-based chromoendoscopy for diagnosis and surveillance in inflammatory bowel disease. Aliment Pharmacol Ther 38:1198–1208
59. Bessissow T, Bisschops R (2013) Advanced endoscopic imaging for dysplasia surveillance in ulcerative colitis. Expert Rev Gastroenterol Hepatol 7:57–67
60. Rutter MD, Saunders BP, Schofield G et al (2004) Pancolonic indigo carmine dye spraying for the detection of dysplasia in ulcerative colitis. Gut 53:256–260
61. Kiesslich R, Goetz M, Lammersdorf K et al (2007) Chromoscopy-guided endomicroscopy increases the diagnostic yield of intraepithelial neoplasia in ulcerative colitis. Gastroenterology 132:874–882
62. Marion JF, Waye JD, Present DH et al (2008) Chromoendoscopy-targeted biopsies are superior to standard colonoscopic surveillance for detecting dysplasia in inflammatory bowel disease patients: a prospective endoscopic trial. Am J Gastroenterol 103:2342–2349
63. Kudo S, Rubio CA, Teixeira CR et al (2001) Pit pattern in colorectal neoplasia: endoscopic magnifying view. Endoscopy 33:367–373
64. Kiesslich R, Fritsch J, Holtmann M et al (2003) Methylene blue-aided chromoendoscopy for the detection of intraepithelial neoplasia and colon cancer in ulcerative colitis. Gastroenterology 124:880–888
65. Rutter MD, Saunders BP, Wilkinson KH et al (2004) Most dysplasia in ulcerative colitis is visible at colonoscopy. Gastrointest Endosc 60:334–339
66. Hurlstone DP, Sanders DS, Lobo AJ et al (2005) Indigo carmine-assisted high-magnification chromoscopic colonoscopy for the detection and characterisation of intraepithelial neoplasia in ulcerative colitis: a prospective evaluation. Endoscopy 37:1186–1192
67. Dekker E, van den Broek FJ, Reitsma JB et al (2007) Narrow-band imaging compared with conventional colonoscopy for the detection of dysplasia in patients with longstanding ulcerative colitis. Endoscopy 39:216–221
68. Matsumoto T, Moriyama T, Yao T et al (2007) Autofluorescence imaging colonoscopy for the diagnosis of dysplasia in ulcerative colitis. Inflamm Bowel Dis 13:640–641
69. Messmann H, Endlicher E, Freunek G et al (2003) Fluorescence endoscopy for the detection of low and high grade dysplasia in ulcerative colitis using systemic or local 5-aminolaevulinic acid sensitisation. Gut 52:1003–1007
70. Kiesslich R, Neurath MF (2008) What new endoscopic imaging modalities will become important in the diagnosis of IBD? Inflamm Bowel Dis 14(Suppl 2):S172–S176
71. Kiesslich R, Burg J, Vieth M et al (2004) Confocal laser endoscopy for diagnosing intraepithelial neoplasias and colorectal cancer in vivo. Gastroenterology 127:706–713
72. Gono K, Obi T, Yamaguchi M et al (2004) Appearance of enhanced tissue features in narrow-band endoscopic imaging. J Biomed Opt 9:568–577
73. Zabrodsky M, Lukes P, Lukesova E et al (2014) The role of narrow band imaging in the detection of recurrent laryngeal and hypopharyngeal cancer after curative radiotherapy. Biomed Res Int 2014:175398
74. van den Broek FJ, Fockens P, van Eeden S et al (2011) Narrow-band imaging versus high-definition endoscopy for the diagnosis of neoplasia in ulcerative colitis. Endoscopy 43:108–115
75. Ignjatovic A, East JE, Subramanian V et al (2012) Narrow band imaging for detection of dysplasia in colitis: a randomized controlled trial. Am J Gastroenterol 107:885–890
76. Efthymiou M, Allen PB, Taylor AC et al (2013) Chromoendoscopy versus narrow band imaging for colonic surveillance in inflammatory bowel disease. Inflamm Bowel Dis 19:2132–2138
77. Pellise M, Lopez-Ceron M, Rodriguez de Miguel C et al (2011) Narrow-band imaging as an alternative to chromoendoscopy for the detection of dysplasia in long-standing inflammatory bowel disease: a prospective, randomized, crossover study. Gastrointest Endosc 74:840–848

78. Watanabe K, Sogawa M, Yamagami H et al (2011) Endoscopic differential diagnosis between ulcerative colitis-associated neoplasia and sporadic neoplasia in surveillance colonoscopy using narrow band imaging. Dig Endosc 23(Suppl 1):143–149
79. DaCosta RS, Andersson H, Wilson BC (2003) Molecular fluorescence excitation-emission matrices relevant to tissue spectroscopy. Photochem Photobiol 78:384–392
80. DaCosta RS, Wilson BC, Marcon NE (2005) Optical techniques for the endoscopic detection of dysplastic colonic lesions. Curr Opin Gastroenterol 21:70–79
81. van den Broek FJ, Fockens P, van Eeden S et al (2008) Endoscopic tri-modal imaging for surveillance in ulcerative colitis: randomised comparison of high-resolution endoscopy and autofluorescence imaging for neoplasia detection; and evaluation of narrow-band imaging for classification of lesions. Gut 57:1083–1089
82. Peng Q, Warloe T, Berg K et al (1997) 5-Aminolevulinic acid-based photodynamic therapy. Clinical research and future challenges. Cancer 79:2282–2308
83. Gamarra F, Lingk P, Marmarova A et al (2004) 5-Aminolevulinic acid-induced fluorescence in bronchial tumours: dependency on the patterns of tumour invasion. J Photochem Photobiol B 73:35–42
84. Kriegmair M, Baumgartner R, Knuechel R et al (1994) Fluorescence photodetection of neoplastic urothelial lesions following intravesical instillation of 5-aminolevulinic acid. Urology 44:836–841
85. Neumann H, Kiesslich R, Wallace MB et al (2010) Confocal laser endomicroscopy: technical advances and clinical applications. Gastroenterology 139:388–392, 392 e381-382
86. Hurlstone DP, Kiesslich R, Thomson M et al (2008) Confocal chromoscopic endomicroscopy is superior to chromoscopy alone for the detection and characterisation of intraepithelial neoplasia in chronic ulcerative colitis. Gut 57:196–204
87. Morson BC, Pang LS (1967) Rectal biopsy as an aid to cancer control in ulcerative colitis. Gut 8:423–434
88. Blackstone MO, Riddell RH, Rogers BH et al (1981) Dysplasia-associated lesion or mass (DALM) detected by colonoscopy in long-standing ulcerative colitis: an indication for colectomy. Gastroenterology 80:366–374
89. Bernstein CN, Shanahan F, Weinstein WM (1994) Are we telling patients the truth about surveillance colonoscopy in ulcerative colitis? Lancet 343:71–74
90. Dyson JK, Rutter MD (2012) Colorectal cancer in inflammatory bowel disease: what is the real magnitude of the risk? World J Gastroenterol 18:3839–3848
91. Hirai TKT, Kanemitsu Y (2002) Colorectal cancer in patients with inflammatory bowel disease in Japan. Stomach Intestine 37:887–893
92. Mpofu C, Watson AJ, Rhodes JM (2004) Strategies for detecting colon cancer and/or dysplasia in patients with inflammatory bowel disease. Cochrane Database Syst Rev CD000279
93. Collins PD, Mpofu C, Watson AJ et al (2006) Strategies for detecting colon cancer and/or dysplasia in patients with inflammatory bowel disease. Cochrane Database Syst Rev CD000279
94. Karlen P, Kornfeld D, Brostrom O et al (1998) Is colonoscopic surveillance reducing colorectal cancer mortality in ulcerative colitis? A population based case control study. Gut 42:711–714
95. Choi PM, Nugent FW, Schoetz DJ Jr et al (1993) Colonoscopic surveillance reduces mortality from colorectal cancer in ulcerative colitis. Gastroenterology 105:418–424
96. Lashner BA, Kane SV, Hanauer SB (1990) Colon cancer surveillance in chronic ulcerative colitis: historical cohort study. Am J Gastroenterol 85:1083–1087
97. Friedman S, Rubin PH, Bodian C et al (2008) Screening and surveillance colonoscopy in chronic Crohn's colitis: results of a surveillance program spanning 25 years. Clin Gastroenterol Hepatol 6:993–998
98. Itzkowitz SH, Present DH, Crohn's et al (2005) Consensus conference: colorectal cancer screening and surveillance in inflammatory bowel disease. Inflamm Bowel Dis 11:314–321

99. Thomas M, Bienkowski R, Vandermeer TJ et al (2010) Malignant transformation in perianal fistulas of Crohn's disease: a systematic review of literature. J Gastrointest Surg 14:66–73
100. Devon KM, Brown CJ, Burnstein M et al (2009) Cancer of the anus complicating perianal Crohn's disease. Dis Colon Rectum 52:211–216
101. Iesalnieks I, Gaertner WB, Glass H et al (2010) Fistula-associated anal adenocarcinoma in Crohn's disease. Inflamm Bowel Dis 16:1643–1648
102. Odze RD, Goldblum J, Noffsinger A et al (2002) Interobserver variability in the diagnosis of ulcerative colitis-associated dysplasia by telepathology. Mod Pathol 15:379–386
103. Eaden J, Abrams K, McKay H et al (2001) Inter-observer variation between general and specialist gastrointestinal pathologists when grading dysplasia in ulcerative colitis. J Pathol 194:152–157
104. Connell WR, Lennard-Jones JE, Williams CB et al (1994) Factors affecting the outcome of endoscopic surveillance for cancer in ulcerative colitis. Gastroenterology 107:934–944
105. Lim CH, Dixon MF, Vail A et al (2003) Ten year follow up of ulcerative colitis patients with and without low grade dysplasia. Gut 52:1127–1132
106. Lindberg B, Persson B, Veress B et al (1996) Twenty years' colonoscopic surveillance of patients with ulcerative colitis. Detection of dysplastic and malignant transformation. Scand J Gastroenterol 31:1195–1204
107. Eaden J, Abrams K, Ekbom A et al (2000) Colorectal cancer prevention in ulcerative colitis: a case-control study. Aliment Pharmacol Ther 14:145–153

Chapter 5
Molecular Alterations in Inflammatory Colonic Carcinogenesis and Markers for Detecting Colitis-Associated Cancer

Yuji Toiyama, Toshimitsu Araki, Koji Tanaka, Yasuhiko Mohri, and Masato Kusunoki

Abstract The incidence of colorectal neoplasia is higher among patients with long-standing and extensive ulcerative colitis (UC) and Crohn's disease (CD), such as that for these patients surveillance colonoscopy is widely recommended. However, colitis-associated cancer (CAC) is often difficult to detect endoscopically and histologically because of modifications of the mucosal structure by inflammation. Repeated flare-ups of inflammation are believed to promote oncogenic insults to the colonic epithelium. Chronic inflammation and thus the increased turnover of epithelial cells contribute to the development of low-grade and high-grade dysplasia and therefore, over time, CAC. This is a different sequence of tumorigenic events that occurs in the development of sporadic CRC. Although the genetic and epigenetic features that lead to sporadic CRC (chromosomal instability, microsatellite instability, DNA methylation, and microRNAs) also occur in CAC, in the inflamed colonic mucosa, unlike the normal mucosa, these molecular alterations take place before there is any histopathologic evidence of dysplasia and cancer. Recently, several molecular alterations of the nonneoplastic epithelium have been identified in UC patients with neoplasia. These alterations may be promising as markers for identifying patients at high risk of developing CAC.

Keywords Inflammatory bowel disease • Colitis-associated cancer • Carcinogenesis • Molecular alteration • Diagnosis

5.1 Introduction

Patients with long-standing inflammatory bowel disease (IBD), including ulcerative colitis (UC) and Crohn's disease (CD), are at a higher risk than the general population of developing colorectal cancer (CRC). This risk increases with a longer

Y. Toiyama (✉) • T. Araki • K. Tanaka • Y. Mohri • M. Kusunoki
Department of Gastrointestinal and Pediatric Surgery, Division of Reparative Medicine, Institute of Life Sciences, Graduate School of Medicine, Mie University, 2-174 Edobashi, Tsu, Mie 514-8507, Japan
e-mail: ytoi0725@clin.medic.mie-u.ac.jp

M. Kusunoki (ed.), *Colitis-Associated Cancer*, DOI 10.1007/978-4-431-55522-3_5

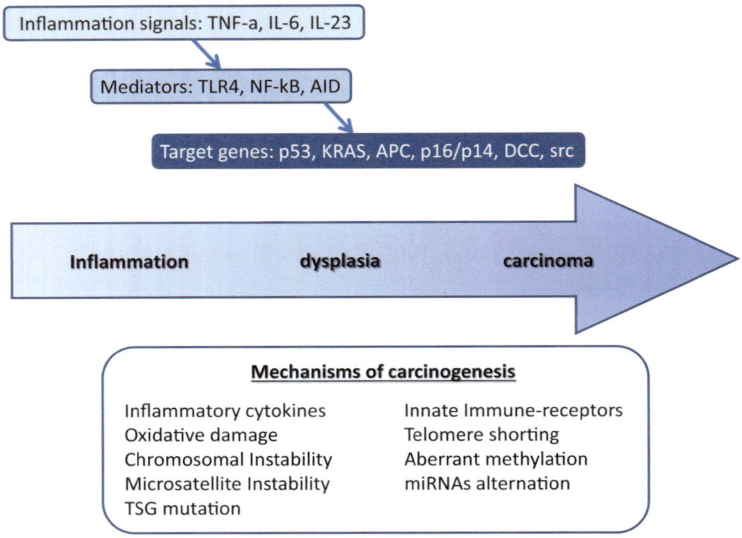

Fig. 5.1 Molecular pathogenesis of colorectal dysplasia and cancer in inflammatory bowel disease. Summary of the molecular signals, mediators, gene targets, and mechanisms implicated in the progression from mucosal inflammation to dysplasia to cancer. Abbreviations: *AID* activation-induced cytidine deaminase, *IL* interleukin, *TLR* Toll-like receptor, *TNF* tumor necrosis factor, *TSG* tumor suppressor gene

duration of colitis, the greater extent of inflammation, a family history of CRC, the severity of bowel inflammation, and a coexistent primary sclerosing cholangitis. The cornerstone for comprehending the development of colitis-associated cancer (CAC) in IBD and hence its early detection is based on an understanding of the molecular pathways of IBD itself. At a molecular level, the pathogenesis of CAC is related to the inflammatory changes, which involve multiple interrelated pathways including: (1) mucosal inflammatory mediators, such as cyclooxygenase-2 (Cox-2), interleukin (IL)-6, IL-10, tumor necrosis factor (TNF)-α, nuclear factor-kB, and chemokines; (2) oxidant stress; (3) changes in the expression of immune receptors on epithelial cells, including Toll-like receptors and Nod1; and (iv) genetic alterations, such as chromosomal and microsatellite instability, hypermethylation, and microRNAs (Fig. 5.1). The aim of this review is to provide an evidence-based approach to the role of chronic inflammatory mechanisms and their molecular basis in the development of CAC. An understanding of the molecular basis of CRC is an important step in the identification of new biomarkers that can help in the early detection of malignancy.

5.2 Inflammation

During inflammation, the destiny of an epithelial cell is determined by the balance between pro- and anti-tumorigenic immune responses. Inflammation participates in the three main stages of carcinogenesis: tumor initiation, tumor promotion, and tumor progression. Tumor initiation defines the process by which a normal cell becomes premalignant. The inflammatory condition, in which the levels of cytokines, chemokines, and reactive oxygen and nitrogen species are increased, induces DNA mutations, epigenetic alterations, and genomic instability, all of which contribute to tumor initiation [1, 2]. Tumor promotion leads to the proliferation of genetically altered cells, which is enhanced by inflammation via the acceleration of anti-apoptosis, proliferation, and angiogenesis [1, 2]. Finally, genetic changes influenced by inflammation advance tumor spread from the primary site to multiple distant sites (metastasis) [1, 2]. Thus, inflammation and malignant tumor formation are closely connected at all stage of tumorigenesis.

Much of the current evidence regarding the inflammatory mediators of CAC comes from murine models, which have provided insights into the carcinogenic process [3]. For example, IL-10-deficient mice develop spontaneous colitis and colonic neoplasms similar to those that occur in patients with CD [4]. Mice can also be treated with the mucosal irritant dextran sulfate sodium (DSS), with or without the mutagenic agent azoxymethane (AOM), which induces damage similar to that seen in UC patients, following a dose-repeated oral administration, colitis, and colonic neoplasm [5–7]. Through animal models, it is now known that inflammatory cytokines, chemokines, cell-surface receptors, and microbiota in the gut play crucial roles in colitis-associated carcinogenesis.

Cytokines exhibit both pro-inflammatory and anti-inflammatory effects, the balance of which plays an important role in CAC [3]. TNF-α, a pro-inflammatory cytokine, is an important mediator of chronic inflammatory disease, including IBD. TNF-α levels are consistently upregulated in the blood and colonic mucosa of patients with IBD [8]. In carcinogenesis, TNF-α acts as a tumor initiator by stimulating the production of reactive oxygen species, which cause oxidative stress and thus DNA damage and mutations and, in turn, tumor promotion, by altering cell proliferation and cell death [9–11]. Consistent with the critical role of TNF-α in chronic inflammation, anti-TNF-α monoclonal antibody biologics, such as infliximab, adalimumab, and certolizumab pegol, have proven to be effective in the treatment of IBD [10]. Furthermore, in an in vivo study using a mouse model of colitis, a monoclonal anti-TNF-α antibody reduced the development of tumors [2]. These results confirm the critical role of TNF-α in chronic inflammation and CAC. The pro-inflammatory cytokine IL-6 mediates a wide variety of inflammation-associated diseases. IL-6 levels are increased in IBD, CRC, and CAC and contribute to CAC development by promoting the survival of neoplastic epithelial cells in the colon [12–15]. Thus, the blockage of IL-6 signaling transduction could be a useful therapeutic system for the treatment of CAC [16]. IL-6 is also involved in promoting the growth and tumorigenesis of colon cancer cells by altering the epigenome, such as silencing of DNA methyltransferase 1 (DNMT1)-mediated tumor suppressor genes [17]. Therefore, IL-6 appears to play a critical role in inflammation-associated carcinogenesis, although the molecular mechanisms are still being elucidated. Another important regulator of the immune response is the anti-inflammatory cytokine IL-10; its function is to block nuclear factor-kappaB (NF-kB) activity and to regulate the Jak-Stat signaling pathway [18, 19]. In addition, IL-10 downregulates TNF-α, vascular endothelial growth factor, and IL-6 production, which may account for its inhibitory effect on the tumor stroma [20]. IL-10 null mice develop spontaneous, generalized colitis and CAC in the presence of enteric bacteria. [21], whereas the administration of IL-10 improves the colitis and reduces tumor development by 50 %, even after colitis establishment [22]. Therefore, an incorrect balance of both pro- and anti-inflammatory cytokines is critical to both inflammation and inflammation-associated carcinogenesis.

Intraluminal bacterial endotoxins, TNF-α, and other pro-inflammatory cytokines act through extracellular receptors such as Toll-like receptors (TLRs) to initiate the phosphorylation cascades that transmit signals to key transcription factors such as NF-kB [23, 24]. TLR-4, which specifically responds to bacterial lipopolysaccharide ligand and is expressed at low levels in normal intestinal mucosa, is upregulated in the mucosa of patients with IBD, in the ileal mucosa of UC patients with pouchitis, in UC-associated CRC, and in colon tumors that develop in the AOM/DSS mouse model [25–27]. By contrast, TLR-4-deficient mice develop fewer and smaller tumors and produce less Cox-2 and prostaglandin E2, both of which mediate colorectal tumorigenesis. Conversely, mice deficient in the cytoplasmic immune receptor Nod1 and treated with AOM/DSS develop more severe colitis and larger tumors in the colonic mucosa compared to controls [28]. Taken together, these observations show that interactions between commensal bacterial components, elements of the innate immune response, and inflammation-induced tumorigenesis [29] are important for the initiation and maintenance of both chronic inflammation and tumor progression, through processes that involve NF-kB-regulated cytokines, chemokines, angiogenic factors, anti-apoptotic factors, and matrix proteases.

The mechanisms by which inflammatory cytokines promote the epithelial DNA mutations necessary for the initiation of neoplasia remain largely undefined. However, a potential mechanism has recently emerged from the study of activation-induced cytidine deaminase (AID), an enzyme that under physiologic conditions regulates class switching and somatic hypermutation in the immunoglobulin genes of activated B cells. AID induction by pro-inflammatory cytokines in human colon cancer cell lines was shown to lead to the accumulation of mutations in the tumor suppressor gene p53 [30]. AID is overexpressed in both neoplastic and nonneoplastic colonic epithelium from patients with IBD, as well as in some sporadic colon cancers. Therefore, this mechanism may account for the production of other potentially carcinogenic mutations in colonic epithelial cells in response to the overexpression of pro-inflammatory cytokines.

5.3 Oxidative Stress

Inflammation gives rise to colonic carcinogenesis by generating oxidative stress. IBD has been viewed as an oxyradical overload disease, in which long-standing inflammation increases the risk of malignant tumors [31]. Oxidative stress causes cellular damage that contributes to the pathogenesis of the colitis itself and to colon carcinogenesis. The initiation of tumor formation in chronic inflammatory tissue might be induced by reactive oxygen and nitrogen species (RONS), which are released by cells of the innate immune system. The inflamed colonic mucosa of patients with active IBD-associated colitis is characterized by the increased expression of nitric oxide synthase (NOS) and RONS [32–34]. Additionally, McKenzie et al. demonstrated the oxidation of thiols in the active site of glyceraldehyde-3-phosphate dehydrogenase, with subsequent inhibition of enzyme activity, in colonic epithelial cells from the inflamed mucosa of patients with IBD but not from paired samples of non-inflamed mucosa [35]. Furthermore, measurements of 8-hydroxydeoxyguanosine in mucosal biopsies from patients with UC showed that oxidative DNA damage progressively accumulates with the increasing duration of UC, reaching maximal levels in dysplastic lesions. This observation has implications for mutagenic and carcinogenic progression.

There is also evidence regarding the mechanisms of colorectal carcinogenesis induced by oxidative stress. Free radicals affect many metabolic processes, including those that regulate DNA, RNA, proteins, and lipids [31, 36]. When free radicals alter the genes or proteins that maintain homeostasis in intestinal epithelial cells, for example, p53, a dysplastic lesion forms and ultimately CAC. Hussain and coworkers [37] compared mutations of p53 in biopsy samples collected from the inflamed colonic mucosa of UC patients and from the normal mucosa of individuals without UC. The majority of the UC samples had a high frequency of p53 mutations compared with the control. In addition, these mutations were found only in inflamed not in non-inflamed mucosa. Another group showed that hydrogen peroxide inactivated the mismatch repair (MMR) system in colorectal cancer cell lines, apparently by damaging the protein complexes responsible for DNA repair [38] and causing microsatellite instability (MSI). In fact, MSI has been detected in the chronic inflammatory mucosa of UC patients, even in those with short disease duration, before the risk of dysplasia or CAC increases [39]. By contrast, MSI was not found in the colonic mucosa of healthy controls or that of patients with benign colitis or that of patients with CD [39, 40]. Thus, only a specific type of UC-induced colitis appears to cause MSI.

Several animal models have demonstrated that RONS participate in colitis-induced carcinogenesis. The application of peroxynitrite to the rat rectum was shown to cause colonic inflammation [41]. Scavengers of oxygen radicals (such as superoxide dismutase), catalase, and NOS inhibitors attenuate inflammation of the colon in animal models of chemically induced colonic injury [42]. Likewise, mice with inducible knockout of NOS develop attenuated colitis in response to injury [43], and APCmin/+ mice, carrying a mutation in the adenomatous polyposis coli gene that causes multiple intestinal adenomas, developed fewer adenomas when they were crossed with mice carrying an inducible knockout of NOS or given an inducible NOS inhibitor. Although APCmin/+ mice are not considered to be models of colon cancers that arise from colitis, these data support the concept that oxidative stress promotes colon carcinogenesis. The fact that mice deficient in glutathione peroxidase enzymes develop inflammation and cancer of the small and large intestines also supports a model in which antioxidant pathways prevent the transition of inflammation to neoplasia.

5.4 Genetic Instability

Genetic instability can be divided into two clinically distinct forms, both of which have been extensively studied in CRC: chromosomal instability (CIN) and MSI [44]. CIN and MSI are detected with the same frequency in CAC (85 % CIN, 15 % MSI) as in sporadic CRC [45]. CIN is manifested by genomic alterations that affect large DNA segments, resulting in aneuploidy, translocations, deletions, gene copy amplifications, and telomere shortening. It is typically associated with the progressive accumulation of mutations in onco-suppressor genes (APC, p53) and oncogenes (KRAS). MSI can be preceded by the alternation/inactivation of DNA repair mechanisms, including nucleotide excision repair, base excision repair, and MMR [46]. Furthermore, besides the many genetic contributions to CIN and MSI, epigenetic elements can affect tumor initiation, proliferation, and metastasis. In particular, the hypermethylation of onco-suppressor DNA promoter regions and microRNAs are major epigenetic mechanisms of gene silencing in colorectal carcinogenesis [47].

5.4.1 Chromosomal Instability

The extent and types of CIN associated with IBD-related dysplasia and CAC have been evaluated by comparative genomic hybridization, fluorescent in situ hybridization (FISH), flow cytometry, and DNA fingerprinting. CIN in IBD, in addition to its similar frequency to CIN in sporadic carcinogenesis, also affects many of the same loci and results in similar mean numbers of chromosomal alterations per case [45, 48]. An important distinction, however, is that CIN in UC is distributed broadly, involving even mucosa that is negative for and remote from dysplasia, whereas in sporadic CRC it is restricted to tumor tissues [45, 49, 50]. Chromosomal alterations therefore appear to occur early in the course of IBD-related neoplastic progression and prior to the histologic features of dysplasia. CIN is typically absent in patients with UC who do not also harbor dysplasia or CAC. Thus, the presence or absence of CIN in nonneoplastic mucosa has been advanced as a marker enabling patients to be stratified into distinct categories of progressors and non-progressors, respectively [45, 49, 51–53]. Progressors have an earlier onset and longer duration of disease [54]. Recently, the FISH-based detection of combined alterations in four key chromosomes in nonneoplastic mucosa was reported to be 100 % sensitive and 92 % specific in distinguishing progressors from non-progressors, suggesting the application of this method to improve surveillance [55]. One proposed mechanism by which chronic inflammation could lead to CIN involves accelerated telomere shortening. The telomeres of colonic epithelial cells from patients with UC are shorter than those of the colonic epithelial cells of healthy controls. This difference is attributable to the faster cell turnover, increased replication, and increased oxidative damage that result from repeated cycles of injury and regeneration [56, 57]. Telomere shortening in turn correlates with CIN, as reflected by the higher rates of chromosomal arm and centromere loss and the higher frequency of anaphase bridges in the colonic epithelium of patients with UC who have dysplasia or CAC but not in that of controls [53]. Telomere shortening beyond a critical point is associated with aging as well as growth arrest, through replicative senescence when DNA damage checkpoints are intact, but through chromosomal damage, such as breaks and end-to-end fusions, when these checkpoints are defective [58, 59]. Thus, telomere shortening could facilitate CIN, provided that DNA damage checkpoints are somehow also inactivated through mutations of checkpoint genes such as p53. The rates of telomere shortening in the colonic epithelial cells of patients with UC are double those seen in healthy controls and occur mostly during the first 8 years of disease, the time frame when the risk of CRC begins to become clinically significant [57].

Aneuploidy occurs in approximately 33 % of patients with long-standing UC, in 20–50 % of dysplastic lesions, and in 50–90 % of cancers [60]. Regions of aneuploidy in the large bowel of UC patients are frequently those exhibiting dysplasia. Since aneuploidy precedes the appearance of histologic changes, it may be a useful marker of developing neoplastic lesions in UC patients. Despite the utility of flow cytometry in assessing aneuploidy in patients with IBD, it is not widely available and thus cannot be universally applied in the follow-up of patients with long-standing UC.

The timing and frequency of DNA mutation differs in CAC vs. sporadic CRC (Fig. 5.2). Loss of APC function, an early event in the progression of sporadic CRC, is less frequent and usually occurs at the late stage of CAC development [61–63]. APC mutations are rarely, if ever, detected in cells of the colitic mucosa that are negative or indefinite for dysplasia, and <14 % of tissues with low-grade dysplasia or CAC have mutations in APC [61, 62, 64]. Likewise, allelic deletion of APC occurs in <33 % of CAC cases [64]. Loss of p53 function is an important step in CAC progression, and allelic deletion of p53 is observed in 50–85 % of CACs [65, 66]. Loss of heterozygosity (LOH) at p53, which correlates with malignant progression, was detected in 6 % of biopsy samples without dysplasia, 9 % with indefinite dysplasia, 33 % with low-grade dysplasia, 63 % with high-grade dysplasia, and 85 % with CAC [65]. Mutations in p53 are found in the colon tissue of patients with colitis and often in mucosa that is nonneoplastic or only indefinite for dysplasia [65–67]. In carefully mapped colectomy specimens, p53 mutations

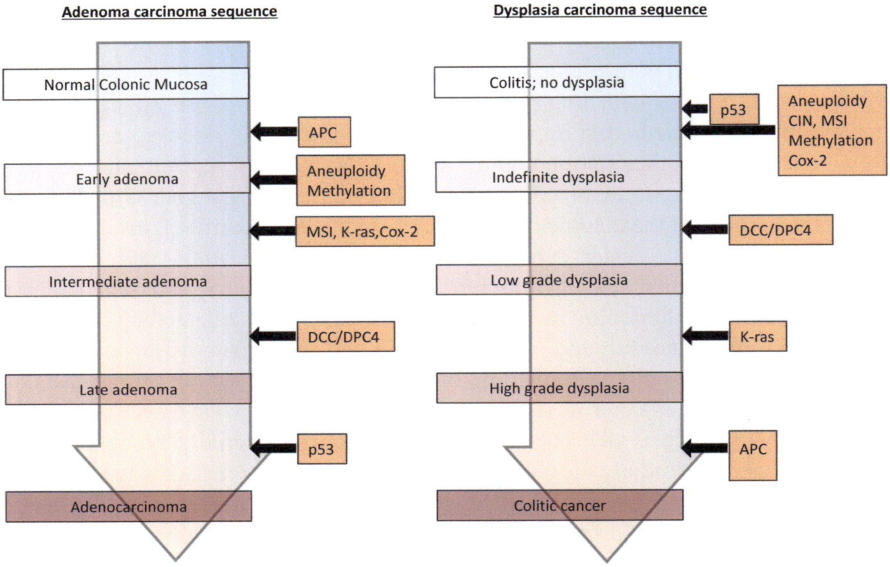

Fig. 5.2 Comparison of the molecular alterations in sporadic colon cancer (*left*) and colitis-associated colorectal cancer (*right*). There are similarities between the two pathways, including the development of chromosomal instability, microsatellite instability, DNA methylation, activation of the KRAS oncogene and of cyclo-oxygenase (Cox)-2, and mutation and the eventual loss of heterozygosity of p53, the adenomatous polyposis coli (APC) gene, and the deleted in colorectal carcinoma (DCC) genes DCC/DPC4. However, the frequency and sequence of these events differ between the pathways

were shown to occur early in tumorigenesis, before aneuploidy [66, 67]. In fact, mutations were found in inflamed mucosa from >50 % of UC patients who did not have CAC, indicating that chronic inflammation caused these mutations [37]. Mutations of the KRAS proto-oncogene, present in 40–60 % of sporadic CRCs, are probably an early event in these cancers [68], whereas they occur at a lower but significant frequency (24 %) in CAC [69]. Thus, KRAS mutations probably play a significant role in the later stage of CAC. The tumor suppressor gene Rb is often mutated or lost in epithelial tumors. In UC-associated carcinogenesis, Rb LOH is present in 20 % of dysplasia and 30 % of CAC specimens [70]. Finally, losses at chromosome 18q are relatively rare events in the sequence of dysplasia → carcinoma in UC. LOH of 18q, the site of the deleted in colorectal carcinoma gene, was observed in 12 % of CACs and 33 % of dysplasias but not in nonneoplastic lesions or inflamed mucosa [71].

5.4.2 Microsatellite Instability

Microsatellites are short repetitive sequences (one to five nucleotides) of DNA that are randomly distributed throughout the whole genome. MSI involves the loss of function of several genes (hMSH2, hMLH1, hPMS1, hPMS2, hMSH6, and hMLH3) that repair DNA base-pair mismatches. DNA MMR deficiency results in a strong mutator phenotype and MSI [72]. The stability of these sequences is a good measure of the general integrity of the genome. MSI reflects a gain or loss of repeat units in a germline microsatellite allele, consistent with the clonal expansion that is typical of cancer. UC-associated carcinogenesis can also be associated with MSI. A high rate of MSI in long-standing UC is probably related to the genomic instability produced by repeated inflammatory stimulation, and the influence of inflammation has been evaluated in estimates of MSI in UC [73]. Indeed, although the molecular mechanisms involved in the increased risk of CAC in UC are for the most part still unclear, many appear to be related to MSI [39]. The prevailing hypothesis is that the overproduction of free radicals overwhelms the ability of the cell to repair oxidative DNA damage prior to replication [39, 74]. Alternatively, prolonged and repeated oxidative insults may directly inactivate DNA MMR genes [38]. One study reported that half of UC mucosal samples with high MSI exhibit MLH1 hypermethylation [75]. However, in contrast to colon cancer in patients with hereditary non-polyposis, there is little evidence for MMR defects as a cause of MSI in UC [76, 77]. A recent report described the adaptive increased activity of 3-methyladenine DNA glycosylase (AAG) and apurinic endonuclease (APE1) in areas of the UC colon undergoing active inflammation [78]. This imbalanced increase appeared to be associated with the MSI characteristic of UC. These data were consistent with a possible novel mechanism by which the colonic cells of patients with chronic colonic inflammation acquire MSI. In UC patients, areas of the colonic epithelium with active inflammation exhibited increased AAG and APE1 enzyme activity; the largest increases and imbalances occurred in areas with inflammation as well as MSI. These observations suggest that the adaptive imbalanced increase in these enzymes has DNA-damaging effects and contributes to carcinogenesis in the chronically inflamed colon [78].

5.4.3 Aberrant DNA Methylation

Epigenetics, which includes histone modifications and DNA methylation, alters gene expression without changing the DNA sequence and can be transmitted to daughter cells. There is also significant cross talk between histone modifications and DNA methylation, both of which are highly dysregulated in many diseases, particularly in cancer [79, 80]. Epigenetic alterations are observed during inflammation and inflammation-associated carcinogenesis [81, 82]. DNA methylation involves the addition of a methyl group to the fifth carbon position in the pyrimidine ring of cytosine located in the context of CpG dinucleotides. It is one of the most well-studied epigenetic processes and is maintained during replication by the enzyme DNMT1, whereas de novo DNA methylation is believed to be mediated by DNMT3A and DNMT3B. However, there is functional overlap between DNMT1, DNMT3A, and DNMT3B [83–85].

DNA methylation contributes to the development and progression of CAC. Methylation of CpG islands in several genes precedes dysplasia and can be detected throughout the mucosa of patients with UC [86]. Among CAC tissues from UC patients, hMLH1 hypermethylation was recognized in six of 13 specimens with high levels of MSI, one of six with low levels of MSI, and four of 27 without MSI [75], suggesting that methylation induces MSI. The attenuated expression of the cell cycle inhibitor gene p16INK4a is associated with sporadic CRC; p16INK4a is also frequently hypermethylated in neoplastic tissues from UC patients. Approximately 10 % of nonneoplastic lesions have hypermethylation of the p16 promoter; the rate increases with higher grades of dysplasia, reaching 100 % in CAC [87]. Additionally, p14ARF, an indirect regulator of p53, is encoded by the same gene as p16INK4a. Loss of expression of p14ARF by hypermethylation is frequently observed in the mucosa of UC patients. In one study, it was detected in 50 % of CAC, 33 % of dysplastic, and 60 % of nonneoplastic mucosal samples collected from UC patients compared with 3.7 % of normal colonic mucosa samples [88]. Another group investigated the methylation status of ten genes [p16, p14, runt-related transcript factor-3 (RUNX3), Cox-2, E-cadherin, methylated-in-tumor-1 (MINT1), MINT31, HPP1, estrogen receptor, and SLC5A8] in tissue samples from CAC and in nonneoplastic colonic mucosa from UC patients with and without neoplasia [89]. Methylation of the promoters of RUNX3, MINT1, and COX-2 was determined and suggests the use of these genes as biomarkers of the presence of CAC in patients with UC. Kuester et al. [90] demonstrated the hypermethylation of death-associated protein kinase (DAPK), a proapoptotic protein implicated in various apoptotic cascades, in UC-associated carcinogenesis in patients with long-standing disease. They also observed the overexpression of DAPK in inflamed colonic epithelium [90], indicative of a protective role for this protein. Thus, the inactivation of DAPK, mediated by promoter hypermethylation, might contribute to the accumulation of UC epithelial cells with genomic damage in response to inflammation and thus to the initiation of carcinogenesis and CAC.

The increasing evidence of inflammation-associated carcinogenesis includes a role for the key mediators of inflammation-induced DNA methylation: oxidative stress and increased levels of the pro-inflammatory cytokines, including IL-6, IL-β, TNF-α, and interferon-ɣ [17, 91–93]. The mechanisms by which these pro-inflammatory mediators alter DNA methylation during inflammation are not completely understood, but recent research has provided several insights. First, IL-6, the expression of which is increased during CAC, stabilizes DNMT1 protein levels in human colon cancer epithelial cells [17]. Second, interferon-ɣ was shown to increase nuclear 5'methylcytidine in human intestinal epithelial cell cultures by increasing DNMT3B mRNA levels [91]. Third, in an animal model of colitis, IL-1β expression was concordant with methylation induction, a phenomenon that is also observed in *Helicobacter pylori* infection, in which increases in IL-1β and TNF-α levels occur in parallel with the temporal changes in methylation levels [93, 94]. Finally, in a colon cancer cell line exposed to oxidative stress, DNMT1 and repressive factors were recruited to GC-rich regions of the genome [92]. These findings suggest that factors produced during inflammation alter mediators of DNA methylation. Thus, the aberrant DNA methylation patterns, rather than being a response to chromosomal insult, may in themselves promote an inflammatory environment. This is supported by a mouse model of colitis, in which aberrant DNA methylation occurred in the absence of macroscopic tumors and gradually increased until tumors developed [94].

According to this scenario, the duration of inflammation is an important factor in aberrant DNA methylation, which is consistent with the duration of IBD being a risk factor for the development of CAC. Whether the inflammation-induced increase in DNA methylation is targeted to specific regions of the genome or affects the genome as a whole remains to be determined.

5.4.4 MicroRNA Alterations

MicroRNAs (miRNAs) are 19–24 nucleotides long and serve as major regulators of gene expression, by targeting mRNAs post-transcriptionally [95]. Important roles for miRNAs have been confirmed in cellular differentiation, development, proliferation, and apoptosis. However, in cancer, these processes are deregulated, which implies that miRNAs are involved in carcinogenesis, perhaps at the tumor initiation and progression stages [96].

Indeed, increasing evidence suggests that miRNAs are involved in the carcinogenesis underlying CAC. Ludwig et al. [97] reported the upregulation of miR-21 in IBD-associated dysplastic lesions but not in tissues from patients with active IBD. The increase in miR-21 correlated inversely with the expression of PDCD4, a newly characterized tumor suppressor gene. Olaru et al. [98, 99] found that miR-224 and miR-31 expression increased successively at each stage of IBD progression, from non-inflamed to inflamed nonneoplastic, dysplastic, and finally cancerous mucosa. Both miR-224 and miR-31 levels could accurately discriminate normal or chronically inflamed IBD tissues from cancers. The authors also showed that miR-224 was involved in cell cycle regulation by targeting p21 and that miR-31, by targeting the negative repressor of hypoxia-inducible factor 1, regulated tumor angiogenesis, which would link both of these miRNAs to IBD-associated carcinogenesis.

In general, tumor-specific miRNA expression profiles are more informative and discriminatory than mRNA profiles. Furthermore, circulating miRNAs are highly resistant to RNase activity, unlike mRNA [100], which recommends their use as noninvasive biomarkers in the diagnosis of CAC. However, miRNA-based markers that confidently identify UC patients at increased risk of neoplasia have yet to be developed.

5.5 Molecular Markers to Identify the Risk of Neoplasia in UC Patients

CAC is a major cause of mortality in patients with UC [101, 102], such that diagnosis at an early or precancerous stage is crucial. A predisposition to colorectal neoplasia in UC is generally considered to depend on the diagnosis of UC at a young age and the presence of extensive colitis [103]. The prevalence of CAC in patients with UC is 8 % at 20 years after the initial UC diagnosis and increases to 18 % at 30 years [104]. Thus, surveillance colonoscopy with multiple random biopsies has been widely recommended for patients with long-standing and extensive UC [105]. However, because CAC is often difficult to detect endoscopically and its discrimination from inflammatory regenerative epithelium is histologically challenging, whether conventional surveillance colonoscopy is effective for the early detection of CAC remains a matter of contention. In addition, recent analysis demonstrated that the low yield and lack of clinical consequences from random biopsies in this high-risk population raise questions about the necessity and cost-effectiveness of routine random biopsy during UC surveillance [106]. Consequently, more accurate diagnostic modalities, such as chromoendoscopy and magnifying endoscopy, to identify potential sites of neoplasia in a nonneoplastic inflamed epithelium, together with analysis of p53 alterations, to distinguish neoplastic lesions from regenerative epithelium, have been evaluated [107, 108]. However, the labor-intensive nature and expense of these adjunctive modalities preclude their use in the surveillance of all UC patients with long-standing and extensive colitis. Rather, within this subgroup of patients, the ability to distinguish those who are at low vs. high risk of colorectal neoplasia would allow physicians to identify patients most likely to benefit from these more extensive screening methods.

5.5.1 Molecular Changes in the Nonneoplastic Mucosa in UC

The nonneoplastic mucosa of UC patients with CAC exhibits several molecular alterations (CIN, MSI, DNA aneuploidy, DNA methylation, telomere shortening, and gene expression), collectively referred to as a "field effect." These alterations in the nonneoplastic UC mucosa may be promising biomarkers that allow the identification of UC patients at high risk of CAC.

5.5.2 Utility of Age-Related Methylation in Identifying CAC

In most human cancers, aberrant hypermethylation of promoter CpG islands, leading to the inactivation of key tumor suppressor genes, is a frequent and early step in tumorigenesis. In CRC, this epigenetic alteration is associated with two distinct subsets of genes: those that display a cancer-restricted methylation pattern (type C) and those that become methylated during aging (type A) [109]. Issa et al. [110] showed that the estrogen receptor (ER) of the normal colorectal mucosa becomes increasingly methylated with age and that hypermethylation of the ER gene is seen in most cases of sporadic CRC. Thus, age-related methylation may be an important contributor to the acquired predisposition to colorectal neoplasia and together with cancer-restricted methylation may be a feature of chronic inflammation-associated disease, including UC.

Issa et al. [86] were the first to demonstrate that the ER, MYOD, and CSPG2 genes and exon 1 of the p16 gene, all of which undergo age-related methylation in the colorectal mucosa, are intensively methylated in the high-grade dysplasia/CAC tissues of UC patients. Furthermore, they showed that these genes were also highly methylated in the nonneoplastic mucosa of these same UC patients. Accordingly, they proposed the use of age-related methylation as a molecular marker to identify UC patients at increased risk of developing dysplasia/CAC. This approach received support from another group that elegantly demonstrated high levels of ER gene methylation not only in regions of dysplasia/CAC but also in other regions widely scattered throughout the colorectum. The implication of the latter result is that analysis of a single biopsy sample (e.g., rectal biopsy) may suffice to identify higher-risk patients and that a large number of biopsy samples and total colonoscopy may not always be necessary [111, 112].

5.5.3 *Methylation of the Putative Promoter Regions of miRNAs as a Marker of CAC in UC Patients*

In an attempt to clarify whether age-related DNA methylation in nonneoplastic epithelium is an indicator of an increased risk for CAC, we selected miR-124, miR-137, and miR-34b/c as candidate genes, since their methylation is associated with increasing age and a field effect has been reported in the uninvolved colonic mucosa of patients with sporadic CRC [113–117]. We hypothesized that aberrant hypermethylation of the genes encoding these specific miRNAs in the normal, aging colorectal epithelium is an early event in CAC. Our systematic evaluation demonstrated the feasibility of using the methylation status of the miR-124, miR-137, and miR-34b/c genes as a promising biomarker in UC-associated neoplasia. When these biomarkers are used alone or in conjunction with the current guidelines for the diagnosis of UC-associated neoplasia, many of the current clinical challenges for managing these patients could be overcome. More importantly, the analysis of these biomarkers from a single rectal biopsy specimen has robust predictive potential in identifying UC patients at high risk for neoplasia elsewhere in the colorectum [118].

5.6 Conclusions and Perspectives

This chapter provided a review of the relationship between colonic inflammation and various tumor genetic events leading to CAC. The sequence of events ending in tumor formation is quite different from the events that give rise to the development of sporadic CRC. The early events in CAC involve DNA methylation, which regulates the expression of onco-suppressor genes, as well as mutation of p53, aneuploidy, and MSI. Tumor- and age-dependent methylation also occur in the nonneoplastic mucosa of UC patients with CAC, so-called field effects. A better understanding of the mechanisms for inflammation-induced carcinogenesis could identify IBD patients at high risk for CAC.

References

1. Karin M, Greten FR (2005) NF-kappaB: linking inflammation and immunity to cancer development and progression. Nat Rev Immunol 5(10):749–759, doi:nri1703 [pii] 10.1038/nri1703
2. Grivennikov SI, Greten FR, Karin M (2010) Immunity, inflammation, and cancer. Cell 140 (6):883–899, doi:S0092-8674(10)00060-7 [pii] 10.1016/j.cell.2010.01.025
3. Kanneganti M, Mino-Kenudson M, Mizoguchi E (2011) Animal models of colitis-associated carcinogenesis. J Biomed Biotechnol 2011:342637. doi:10.1155/2011/342637
4. Sturlan S, Oberhuber G, Beinhauer BG, Tichy B, Kappel S, Wang J, Rogy MA (2001) Interleukin-10-deficient mice and inflammatory bowel disease associated cancer development. Carcinogenesis 22(4):665–671
5. Cooper HS, Murthy S, Kido K, Yoshitake H, Flanigan A (2000) Dysplasia and cancer in the dextran sulfate sodium mouse colitis model. Relevance to colitis-associated neoplasia in the human: a study of histopathology, B-catenin and p53 expression and the role of inflammation. Carcinogenesis 21(4):757–768
6. Okayasu I, Yamada M, Mikami T, Yoshida T, Kanno J, Ohkusa T (2002) Dysplasia and carcinoma development in a repeated dextran sulfate sodium-induced colitis model. J Gastroenterol Hepatol 17(10):1078–1083, doi:2853 [pii]
7. Tanaka T, Kohno H, Suzuki R, Yamada Y, Sugie S, Mori H (2003) A novel inflammation-related mouse colon carcinogenesis model induced by azoxymethane and dextran sodium sulfate. Cancer Sci 94(11):965–973
8. Noguchi M, Hiwatashi N, Liu Z, Toyota T (1998) Secretion imbalance between tumour necrosis factor and its inhibitor in inflammatory bowel disease. Gut 43(2):203–209
9. Di Girolamo N, Visvanathan K, Lloyd A, Wakefield D (1997) Expression of TNF-alpha by human plasma cells in chronic inflammation. J Leukoc Biol 61(6):667–678
10. Wallis RS (2008) Tumour necrosis factor antagonists: structure, function, and tuberculosis risks. Lancet Infect Dis 8(10):601–611, doi:S1473-3099(08)70227-5 [pii] 10.1016/S1473-3099(08)70227-5
11. Szlosarek P, Charles KA, Balkwill FR (2006) Tumour necrosis factor-alpha as a tumour promoter. Eur J Cancer 42(6):745–750, doi:S0959-8049(06)00070-0 [pii] 10.1016/j.ejca.2006.01.012
12. Bromberg J, Wang TC (2009) Inflammation and cancer: IL-6 and STAT3 complete the link. Cancer Cell 15(2):79–80, doi:S1535-6108(09)00006-3 [pii] 10.1016/j.ccr.2009.01.009
13. Bollrath J, Phesse TJ, von Burstin VA, Putoczki T, Bennecke M, Bateman T, Nebelsiek T, Lundgren-May T, Canli O, Schwitalla S, Matthews V, Schmid RM, Kirchner T, Arkan MC,

Ernst M, Greten FR (2009) gp130-mediated Stat3 activation in enterocytes regulates cell survival and cell-cycle progression during colitis-associated tumorigenesis. Cancer Cell 15 (2):91–102, doi:S1535-6108(09)00003-8 [pii] 10.1016/j.ccr.2009.01.002

14. Esfandi F, Mohammadzadeh Ghobadloo S, Basati G (2006) Interleukin-6 level in patients with colorectal cancer. Cancer Lett 244(1):76–78, doi:S0304-3835(05)01052-9 [pii] 10.1016/j.canlet.2005.12.003
15. Li Y, de Haar C, Chen M, Deuring J, Gerrits MM, Smits R, Xia B, Kuipers EJ, van der Woude CJ (2010) Disease-related expression of the IL6/STAT3/SOCS3 signalling pathway in ulcerative colitis and ulcerative colitis-related carcinogenesis. Gut 59(2):227–235, doi: gut.2009.184176 [pii] 10.1136/gut.2009.184176
16. Matsumoto S, Hara T, Mitsuyama K, Yamamoto M, Tsuruta O, Sata M, Scheller J, Rose-John S, Kado S, Takada T (2010) Essential roles of IL-6 trans-signaling in colonic epithelial cells, induced by the IL-6/soluble-IL-6 receptor derived from lamina propria macrophages, on the development of colitis-associated premalignant cancer in a murine model. J Immunol 184(3):1543–1551, doi:jimmunol.0801217 [pii] 10.4049/jimmunol.0801217
17. Foran E, Garrity-Park MM, Mureau C, Newell J, Smyrk TC, Limburg PJ, Egan LJ (2010) Upregulation of DNA methyltransferase-mediated gene silencing, anchorage-independent growth, and migration of colon cancer cells by interleukin-6. Mol Cancer Res 8(4):471–481, doi: 1541-7786.MCR-09-0496 [pii] 10.1158/1541-7786.MCR-09-0496
18. Schottelius AJ, Mayo MW, Sartor RB, Baldwin AS Jr (1999) Interleukin-10 signaling blocks inhibitor of kappaB kinase activity and nuclear factor kappaB DNA binding. J Biol Chem 274 (45):31868–31874
19. Hoentjen F, Sartor RB, Ozaki M, Jobin C (2005) STAT3 regulates NF-kappaB recruitment to the IL-12p40 promoter in dendritic cells. Blood 105(2):689–696, doi:10.1182/blood-2004-04-1309 2004-04-1309 [pii]
20. Huang S, Ullrich SE, Bar-Eli M (1999) Regulation of tumor growth and metastasis by interleukin-10: the melanoma experience. J Interferon Cytokine Res 19(7):697–703. doi:10.1089/107999099313532
21. Moore KW, de Waal Malefyt R, Coffman RL, O'Garra A (2001) Interleukin-10 and the interleukin-10 receptor. Annu Rev Immunol 19:683–765, doi:19/1/683 [pii] 10.1146/annurev.immunol.19.1.683
22. Berg DJ, Davidson N, Kuhn R, Muller W, Menon S, Holland G, Thompson-Snipes L, Leach MW, Rennick D (1996) Enterocolitis and colon cancer in interleukin-10-deficient mice are associated with aberrant cytokine production and CD4(+) TH1-like responses. J Clin Invest 98(4):1010–1020. doi:10.1172/JCI118861
23. Fukata M, Abreu MT (2008) Role of Toll-like receptors in gastrointestinal malignancies. Oncogene 27(2):234–243, doi:1210908 [pii] 10.1038/sj.onc.1210908
24. Maeda S, Omata M (2008) Inflammation and cancer: role of nuclear factor-kappaB activation. Cancer Sci 99(5):836–842, doi:CAS763 [pii] 10.1111/j.1349-7006.2008.00763.x
25. Cario E, Podolsky DK (2000) Differential alteration in intestinal epithelial cell expression of toll-like receptor 3 (TLR3) and TLR4 in inflammatory bowel disease. Infect Immun 68 (12):7010–7017
26. Toiyama Y, Araki T, Yoshiyama S, Hiro J, Miki C, Kusunoki M (2006) The expression patterns of Toll-like receptors in the ileal pouch mucosa of postoperative ulcerative colitis patients. Surg Today 36(3):287–290. doi:10.1007/s00595-005-3144-y
27. Fukata M, Chen A, Vamadevan AS, Cohen J, Breglio K, Krishnareddy S, Hsu D, Xu R, Harpaz N, Dannenberg AJ, Subbaramaiah K, Cooper HS, Itzkowitz SH, Abreu MT (2007) Toll-like receptor-4 promotes the development of colitis-associated colorectal tumors. Gastroenterology 133(6):1869–1881, doi:S0016-5085(07)01649-6 [pii] 10.1053/j.gastro.2007.09.008
28. Chen GY, Shaw MH, Redondo G, Nunez G (2008) The innate immune receptor Nod1 protects the intestine from inflammation-induced tumorigenesis. Cancer Res 68 (24):10060–10067, doi:68/24/10060 [pii] 10.1158/0008-5472.CAN-08-2061

29. Clevers H (2004) At the crossroads of inflammation and cancer. Cell 118(6):671–674, doi:10.1016/j.cell.2004.09.005 S0092867404008347 [pii]
30. Endo Y, Marusawa H, Kou T, Nakase H, Fujii S, Fujimori T, Kinoshita K, Honjo T, Chiba T (2008) Activation-induced cytidine deaminase links between inflammation and the development of colitis-associated colorectal cancers. Gastroenterology 135(3):889–898, 898 e881-883. doi:S0016-5085(08)01325-5 [pii] 10.1053/j.gastro.2008.06.091
31. Hussain SP, Hofseth LJ, Harris CC (2003) Radical causes of cancer. Nat Rev Cancer 3 (4):276–285, doi:10.1038/nrc1046 nrc1046 [pii]
32. Hofseth LJ, Saito S, Hussain SP, Espey MG, Miranda KM, Araki Y, Jhappan C, Higashimoto Y, He P, Linke SP, Quezado MM, Zurer I, Rotter V, Wink DA, Appella E, Harris CC (2003) Nitric oxide-induced cellular stress and p53 activation in chronic inflammation. Proc Natl Acad Sci U S A 100(1):143–148, doi:10.1073/pnas.0237083100 0237083100 [pii]
33. Kimura H, Hokari R, Miura S, Shigematsu T, Hirokawa M, Akiba Y, Kurose I, Higuchi H, Fujimori H, Tsuzuki Y, Serizawa H, Ishii H (1998) Increased expression of an inducible isoform of nitric oxide synthase and the formation of peroxynitrite in colonic mucosa of patients with active ulcerative colitis. Gut 42(2):180–187
34. Rachmilewitz D, Stamler JS, Bachwich D, Karmeli F, Ackerman Z, Podolsky DK (1995) Enhanced colonic nitric oxide generation and nitric oxide synthase activity in ulcerative colitis and Crohn's disease. Gut 36(5):718–723
35. McKenzie SJ, Baker MS, Buffinton GD, Doe WF (1996) Evidence of oxidant-induced injury to epithelial cells during inflammatory bowel disease. J Clin Invest 98(1):136–141. doi:10.1172/JCI118757
36. Marnett LJ (2000) Oxyradicals and DNA damage. Carcinogenesis 21(3):361–370
37. Hussain SP, Amstad P, Raja K, Ambs S, Nagashima M, Bennett WP, Shields PG, Ham AJ, Swenberg JA, Marrogi AJ, Harris CC (2000) Increased p53 mutation load in noncancerous colon tissue from ulcerative colitis: a cancer-prone chronic inflammatory disease. Cancer Res 60(13):3333–3337
38. Chang CL, Marra G, Chauhan DP, Ha HT, Chang DK, Ricciardiello L, Randolph A, Carethers JM, Boland CR (2002) Oxidative stress inactivates the human DNA mismatch repair system. Am J Physiol Cell Physiol 283(1):C148–C154. doi:10.1152/ajpcell.00422.2001
39. Brentnall TA, Crispin DA, Bronner MP, Cherian SP, Hueffed M, Rabinovitch PS, Rubin CE, Haggitt RC, Boland CR (1996) Microsatellite instability in nonneoplastic mucosa from patients with chronic ulcerative colitis. Cancer Res 56(6):1237–1240
40. Noffsinger A, Kretschmer S, Belli J, Fogt F, Fenoglio-Preiser C (2000) Microsatellite instability is uncommon in intestinal mucosa of patients with Crohn's disease. Dig Dis Sci 45(2):378–384
41. Rachmilewitz D, Stamler JS, Karmeli F, Mullins ME, Singel DJ, Loscalzo J, Xavier RJ, Podolsky DK (1993) Peroxynitrite-induced rat colitis--a new model of colonic inflammation. Gastroenterology 105(6):1681–1688, doi:S0016508593003920 [pii]
42. Seril DN, Liao J, Yang GY, Yang CS (2003) Oxidative stress and ulcerative colitis-associated carcinogenesis: studies in humans and animal models. Carcinogenesis 24(3):353–362
43. Ahn B, Ohshima H (2001) Suppression of intestinal polyposis in Apc(Min/+) mice by inhibiting nitric oxide production. Cancer Res 61(23):8357–8360
44. Lengauer C, Kinzler KW, Vogelstein B (1998) Genetic instabilities in human cancers. Nature 396(6712):643–649. doi:10.1038/25292
45. Willenbucher RF, Aust DE, Chang CG, Zelman SJ, Ferrell LD, Moore DH 2nd, Waldman FM (1999) Genomic instability is an early event during the progression pathway of ulcerative-colitis-related neoplasia. Am J Pathol 154(6):1825–1830, doi:S0002-9440(10)65438-7 [pii] 10.1016/S0002-9440(10)65438-7
46. Charames GS, Bapat B (2003) Genomic instability and cancer. Curr Mol Med 3(7):589–596

47. D'Inca R, Cardin R, Benazzato L, Angriman I, Martines D, Sturniolo GC (2004) Oxidative DNA damage in the mucosa of ulcerative colitis increases with disease duration and dysplasia. Inflamm Bowel Dis 10(1):23–27
48. Aust DE, Willenbucher RF, Terdiman JP, Ferrell LD, Chang CG, Moore DH 2nd, Molinaro-Clark A, Baretton GB, Loehrs U, Waldman FM (2000) Chromosomal alterations in ulcerative colitis-related and sporadic colorectal cancers by comparative genomic hybridization. Hum Pathol 31(1):109–114
49. Rabinovitch PS, Dziadon S, Brentnall TA, Emond MJ, Crispin DA, Haggitt RC, Bronner MP (1999) Pancolonic chromosomal instability precedes dysplasia and cancer in ulcerative colitis. Cancer Res 59(20):5148–5153
50. Stoler DL, Chen N, Basik M, Kahlenberg MS, Rodriguez-Bigas MA, Petrelli NJ, Anderson GR (1999) The onset and extent of genomic instability in sporadic colorectal tumor progression. Proc Natl Acad Sci U S A 96(26):15121–15126
51. Chen R, Rabinovitch PS, Crispin DA, Emond MJ, Koprowicz KM, Bronner MP, Brentnall TA (2003) DNA fingerprinting abnormalities can distinguish ulcerative colitis patients with dysplasia and cancer from those who are dysplasia/cancer-free. Am J Pathol 162(2):665–672, doi:S0002-9440(10)63860-6 [pii] 10.1016/S0002-9440(10)63860-6
52. Chen R, Bronner MP, Crispin DA, Rabinovitch PS, Brentnall TA (2005) Characterization of genomic instability in ulcerative colitis neoplasia leads to discovery of putative tumor suppressor regions. Cancer Genet Cytogenet 162(2):99–106, doi:S0165-4608(05)00213-X [pii] 10.1016/j.cancergencyto.2005.04.006
53. O'Sullivan JN, Bronner MP, Brentnall TA, Finley JC, Shen WT, Emerson S, Emond MJ, Gollahon KA, Moskovitz AH, Crispin DA, Potter JD, Rabinovitch PS (2002) Chromosomal instability in ulcerative colitis is related to telomere shortening. Nat Genet 32(2):280–284, doi:10.1038/ng989 ng989 [pii]
54. Brackmann S, Andersen SN, Aamodt G, Roald B, Langmark F, Clausen OP, Aadland E, Fausa O, Rydning A, Vatn MH (2009) Two distinct groups of colorectal cancer in inflammatory bowel disease. Inflamm Bowel Dis 15(1):9–16. doi:10.1002/ibd.20542
55. Bronner MP, O'Sullivan JN, Rabinovitch PS, Crispin DA, Chen L, Emond MJ, Rubin CE, Brentnall TA (2008) Genomic biomarkers to improve ulcerative colitis neoplasia surveillance. Am J Pathol 173(6):1853–1860, doi:S0002-9440(10)61568-4 [pii] 10.2353/ajpath.2008.080250
56. Kinouchi Y, Hiwatashi N, Chida M, Nagashima F, Takagi S, Maekawa H, Toyota T (1998) Telomere shortening in the colonic mucosa of patients with ulcerative colitis. J Gastroenterol 33(3):343–348
57. Risques RA, Lai LA, Brentnall TA, Li L, Feng Z, Gallaher J, Mandelson MT, Potter JD, Bronner MP, Rabinovitch PS (2008) Ulcerative colitis is a disease of accelerated colon aging: evidence from telomere attrition and DNA damage. Gastroenterology 135(2):410–418, doi:S0016-5085(08)00637-9 [pii] 10.1053/j.gastro.2008.04.008
58. Blasco MA (2005) Telomeres and human disease: ageing, cancer and beyond. Nat Rev Genet 6(8):611–622. doi:10.1038/nrg1656
59. Artandi SE, Attardi LD (2005) Pathways connecting telomeres and p53 in senescence, apoptosis, and cancer. Biochem Biophys Res Commun 331(3):881–890, doi:S0006-291X(05)00725-4 [pii] 10.1016/j.bbrc.2005.03.211
60. Rosman-Urbach M, Niv Y, Birk Y, Smirnoff P, Zusman I, Morgenstern S, Schwartz B (2004) A high degree of aneuploidy, loss of p53 gene, and low soluble p53 protein serum levels are detected in ulcerative colitis patients. Dis Colon Rectum 47(3):304–313. doi:10.1007/s10350-003-0048-z
61. Aust DE, Terdiman JP, Willenbucher RF, Chang CG, Molinaro-Clark A, Baretton GB, Loehrs U, Waldman FM (2002) The APC/beta-catenin pathway in ulcerative colitis-related colorectal carcinomas: a mutational analysis. Cancer 94(5):1421–1427, doi:10.1002/cncr.10334 [pii]

62. Redston MS, Papadopoulos N, Caldas C, Kinzler KW, Kern SE (1995) Common occurrence of APC and K-ras gene mutations in the spectrum of colitis-associated neoplasias. Gastroenterology 108(2):383–392, doi:0016-5085(95)90064-0 [pii]
63. Tarmin L, Yin J, Harpaz N, Kozam M, Noordzij J, Antonio LB, Jiang HY, Chan O, Cymes K, Meltzer SJ (1995) Adenomatous polyposis coli gene mutations in ulcerative colitis-associated dysplasias and cancers versus sporadic colon neoplasms. Cancer Res 55 (10):2035–2038
64. Umetani N, Sasaki S, Watanabe T, Shinozaki M, Matsuda K, Ishigami H, Ueda E, Muto T (1999) Genetic alterations in ulcerative colitis-associated neoplasia focusing on APC, K-ras gene and microsatellite instability. Jpn J Cancer Res 90(10):1081–1087, doi: S0910505099801720 [pii]
65. Burmer GC, Rabinovitch PS, Haggitt RC, Crispin DA, Brentnall TA, Kolli VR, Stevens AC, Rubin CE (1992) Neoplastic progression in ulcerative colitis: histology, DNA content, and loss of a p53 allele. Gastroenterology 103(5):1602–1610, doi:S0016508592004360 [pii]
66. Yin J, Harpaz N, Tong Y, Huang Y, Laurin J, Greenwald BD, Hontanosas M, Newkirk C, Meltzer SJ (1993) p53 point mutations in dysplastic and cancerous ulcerative colitis lesions. Gastroenterology 104(6):1633–1639, doi:S0016508593001829 [pii]
67. Brentnall TA, Crispin DA, Rabinovitch PS, Haggitt RC, Rubin CE, Stevens AC, Burmer GC (1994) Mutations in the p53 gene: an early marker of neoplastic progression in ulcerative colitis. Gastroenterology 107(2):369–378, doi:S0016508594002337 [pii]
68. Vogelstein B, Fearon ER, Hamilton SR, Kern SE, Preisinger AC, Leppert M, Nakamura Y, White R, Smits AM, Bos JL (1988) Genetic alterations during colorectal-tumor development. N Engl J Med 319(9):525–532. doi:10.1056/NEJM198809013190901
69. Andersen SN, Lovig T, Clausen OP, Bakka A, Fausa O, Rognum TO (1999) Villous, hypermucinous mucosa in long standing ulcerative colitis shows high frequency of K-ras mutations. Gut 45(5):686–692
70. Greenwald BD, Harpaz N, Yin J, Huang Y, Tong Y, Brown VL, McDaniel T, Newkirk C, Resau JH, Meltzer SJ (1992) Loss of heterozygosity affecting the p53, Rb, and mcc/apc tumor suppressor gene loci in dysplastic and cancerous ulcerative colitis. Cancer Res 52(3):741–745
71. Mikami T, Mitomi H, Hara A, Yanagisawa N, Yoshida T, Tsuruta O, Okayasu I (2000) Decreased expression of CD44, alpha-catenin, and deleted colon carcinoma and altered expression of beta-catenin in ulcerative colitis-associated dysplasia and carcinoma, as compared with sporadic colon neoplasms. Cancer 89(4):733–740, doi:10.1002/1097-0142 (20000815)89:4<733::AID-CNCR3>3.0.CO;2-# [pii]
72. Imai K, Yamamoto H (2008) Carcinogenesis and microsatellite instability: the interrelationship between genetics and epigenetics. Carcinogenesis 29(4):673–680, doi:bgm228 [pii], 10.1093/carcin/bgm228
73. Ishitsuka T, Kashiwagi H, Konishi F (2001) Microsatellite instability in inflamed and neoplastic epithelium in ulcerative colitis. J Clin Pathol 54(7):526–532
74. Loeb KR, Loeb LA (1999) Genetic instability and the mutator phenotype. Studies in ulcerative colitis. Am J Pathol 154(6):1621–1626, doi:S0002-9440(10)65415-6 [pii] 10.1016/S0002-9440(10)65415-6
75. Fleisher AS, Esteller M, Harpaz N, Leytin A, Rashid A, Xu Y, Liang J, Stine OC, Yin J, Zou TT, Abraham JM, Kong D, Wilson KT, James SP, Herman JG, Meltzer SJ (2000) Microsatellite instability in inflammatory bowel disease-associated neoplastic lesions is associated with hypermethylation and diminished expression of the DNA mismatch repair gene, hMLH1. Cancer Res 60(17):4864–4868
76. Cawkwell L, Sutherland F, Murgatroyd H, Jarvis P, Gray S, Cross D, Shepherd N, Day D, Quirke P (2000) Defective hMSH2/hMLH1 protein expression is seen infrequently in ulcerative colitis associated colorectal cancers. Gut 46(3):367–369
77. Noffsinger AE, Belli JM, Fogt F, Fischer J, Goldman H, Fenoglio-Preiser CM (1999) A germline hMSH2 alteration is unrelated to colonic microsatellite instability in patients with ulcerative colitis. Hum Pathol 30(1):8–12

78. Hofseth LJ, Khan MA, Ambrose M, Nikolayeva O, Xu-Welliver M, Kartalou M, Hussain SP, Roth RB, Zhou X, Mechanic LE, Zurer I, Rotter V, Samson LD, Harris CC (2003) The adaptive imbalance in base excision-repair enzymes generates microsatellite instability in chronic inflammation. J Clin Invest 112(12):1887–1894, doi:10.1172/JCI19757 112/12/1887 [pii]
79. Kondo Y (2009) Epigenetic cross-talk between DNA methylation and histone modifications in human cancers. Yonsei Med J 50(4):455–463. doi:10.3349/ymj.2009.50.4.455
80. Fazzari MJ, Greally JM (2010) Introduction to epigenomics and epigenome-wide analysis. Methods Mol Biol 620:243–265. doi:10.1007/978-1-60761-580-4_7
81. Saito S, Kato J, Hiraoka S, Horii J, Suzuki H, Higashi R, Kaji E, Kondo Y, Yamamoto K (2011) DNA methylation of colon mucosa in ulcerative colitis patients: correlation with inflammatory status. Inflamm Bowel Dis 17(9):1955–1965. doi:10.1002/ibd.21573
82. Glauben R, Batra A, Fedke I, Zeitz M, Lehr HA, Leoni F, Mascagni P, Fantuzzi G, Dinarello CA, Siegmund B (2006) Histone hyperacetylation is associated with amelioration of experimental colitis in mice. J Immunol 176(8):5015–5022, doi:176/8/5015 [pii]
83. Fatemi M, Hermann A, Gowher H, Jeltsch A (2002) Dnmt3a and Dnmt1 functionally cooperate during de novo methylation of DNA. Eur J Biochem 269(20):4981–4984, doi:3198 [pii]
84. Jair KW, Bachman KE, Suzuki H, Ting AH, Rhee I, Yen RW, Baylin SB, Schuebel KE (2006) De novo CpG island methylation in human cancer cells. Cancer Res 66(2):682–692, doi:66/2/682 [pii] 10.1158/0008-5472.CAN-05-1980
85. Jeltsch A (2006) On the enzymatic properties of Dnmt1: specificity, processivity, mechanism of linear diffusion and allosteric regulation of the enzyme. Epigenetics 1(2):63–66, doi:2767 [pii]
86. Issa JP, Ahuja N, Toyota M, Bronner MP, Brentnall TA (2001) Accelerated age-related CpG island methylation in ulcerative colitis. Cancer Res 61(9):3573–3577
87. Hsieh CJ, Klump B, Holzmann K, Borchard F, Gregor M, Porschen R (1998) Hypermethylation of the p16INK4a promoter in colectomy specimens of patients with long-standing and extensive ulcerative colitis. Cancer Res 58(17):3942–3945
88. Sato F, Harpaz N, Shibata D, Xu Y, Yin J, Mori Y, Zou TT, Wang S, Desai K, Leytin A, Selaru FM, Abraham JM, Meltzer SJ (2002) Hypermethylation of the p14(ARF) gene in ulcerative colitis-associated colorectal carcinogenesis. Cancer Res 62(4):1148–1151
89. Garrity-Park MM, Loftus EV Jr, Sandborn WJ, Bryant SC, Smyrk TC (2010) Methylation status of genes in non-neoplastic mucosa from patients with ulcerative colitis-associated colorectal cancer. Am J Gastroenterol 105(7):1610–1619, doi:ajg201022 [pii] 10.1038/ajg.2010.22
90. Kuester D, Guenther T, Biesold S, Hartmann A, Bataille F, Ruemmele P, Peters B, Meyer F, Schubert D, Bohr UR, Malfertheiner P, Lippert H, Silver AR, Roessner A, Schneider-Stock R (2010) Aberrant methylation of DAPK in long-standing ulcerative colitis and ulcerative colitis-associated carcinoma. Pathol Res Pract 206(9):616–624, doi:S0344-0338(10)00125-1 [pii] 10.1016/j.prp.2010.05.004
91. Kominsky DJ, Keely S, MacManus CF, Glover LE, Scully M, Collins CB, Bowers BE, Campbell EL, Colgan SP (2011) An endogenously anti-inflammatory role for methylation in mucosal inflammation identified through metabolite profiling. J Immunol 186(11):6505–6514, doi:jimmunol.1002805 [pii] 10.4049/jimmunol.1002805
92. O'Hagan HM, Wang W, Sen S, Destefano Shields C, Lee SS, Zhang YW, Clements EG, Cai Y, Van Neste L, Easwaran H, Casero RA, Sears CL, Baylin SB (2011) Oxidative damage targets complexes containing DNA methyltransferases, SIRT1, and polycomb members to promoter CpG Islands. Cancer Cell 20(5):606–619, doi:S1535-6108(11)00359-X [pii] 10.1016/j.ccr.2011.09.012
93. Niwa T, Tsukamoto T, Toyoda T, Mori A, Tanaka H, Maekita T, Ichinose M, Tatematsu M, Ushijima T (2010) Inflammatory processes triggered by Helicobacter pylori infection cause

aberrant DNA methylation in gastric epithelial cells. Cancer Res 70(4):1430–1440, doi:0008-5472.CAN-09-2755 [pii] 10.1158/0008-5472.CAN-09-2755

94. Katsurano M, Niwa T, Yasui Y, Shigematsu Y, Yamashita S, Takeshima H, Lee MS, Kim YJ, Tanaka T, Ushijima T (2012) Early-stage formation of an epigenetic field defect in a mouse colitis model, and non-essential roles of T- and B-cells in DNA methylation induction. Oncogene 31(3):342–351, doi:onc2011241 [pii] 10.1038/onc.2011.241
95. Lagos-Quintana M, Rauhut R, Lendeckel W, Tuschl T (2001) Identification of novel genes coding for small expressed RNAs. Science 294(5543):853–858, doi:10.1126/science.1064921 294/5543/853 [pii]
96. Taft RJ, Pang KC, Mercer TR, Dinger M, Mattick JS (2010) Non-coding RNAs: regulators of disease. J Pathol 220(2):126–139. doi:10.1002/path.2638
97. Ludwig K, Fassan M, Mescoli C, Pizzi M, Balistreri M, Albertoni L, Pucciarelli S, Scarpa M, Sturniolo GC, Angriman I, Rugge M (2013) PDCD4/miR-21 dysregulation in inflammatory bowel disease-associated carcinogenesis. Virchows Arch 462(1):57–63. doi:10.1007/s00428-012-1345-5
98. Olaru AV, Yamanaka S, Vazquez C, Mori Y, Cheng Y, Abraham JM, Bayless TM, Harpaz N, Selaru FM, Meltzer SJ (2013) MicroRNA-224 negatively regulates p21 expression during late neoplastic progression in inflammatory bowel disease. Inflamm Bowel Dis 19 (3):471–480. doi:10.1097/MIB.0b013e31827e78eb
99. Olaru AV, Selaru FM, Mori Y, Vazquez C, David S, Paun B, Cheng Y, Jin Z, Yang J, Agarwal R, Abraham JM, Dassopoulos T, Harris M, Bayless TM, Kwon J, Harpaz N, Livak F, Meltzer SJ (2011) Dynamic changes in the expression of MicroRNA-31 during inflammatory bowel disease-associated neoplastic transformation. Inflamm Bowel Dis 17 (1):221–231. doi:10.1002/ibd.21359
100. Cortez MA, Bueso-Ramos C, Ferdin J, Lopez-Berestein G, Sood AK, Calin GA (2011) MicroRNAs in body fluids--the mix of hormones and biomarkers. Nat Rev Clin Oncol 8 (8):467–477, doi:nrclinonc.2011.76 [pii] 10.1038/nrclinonc.2011.76
101. Ekbom A, Helmick C, Zack M, Adami HO (1990) Ulcerative colitis and colorectal cancer. A population-based study. N Engl J Med 323(18):1228–1233. doi:10.1056/NEJM199011013231802
102. Langholz E, Munkholm P, Davidsen M, Binder V (1992) Colorectal cancer risk and mortality in patients with ulcerative colitis. Gastroenterology 103(5):1444–1451, doi:S0016508592004347 [pii]
103. Jess T, Rungoe C, Peyrin-Biroulet L (2012) Risk of colorectal cancer in patients with ulcerative colitis: a meta-analysis of population-based cohort studies. Clin Gastroenterol Hepatol 10(6):639–645, doi:S1542-3565(12)00109-7 [pii] 10.1016/j.cgh.2012.01.010
104. Eaden JA, Abrams KR, Mayberry JF (2001) The risk of colorectal cancer in ulcerative colitis: a meta-analysis. Gut 48(4):526–535
105. Winawer S, Fletcher R, Rex D, Bond J, Burt R, Ferrucci J, Ganiats T, Levin T, Woolf S, Johnson D, Kirk L, Litin S, Simmang C (2003) Colorectal cancer screening and surveillance: clinical guidelines and rationale-Update based on new evidence. Gastroenterology 124 (2):544–560, doi:10.1053/gast.2003.50044 S0016508502158951 [pii]
106. van den Broek FJ, Stokkers PC, Reitsma JB, Boltjes RP, Ponsioen CY, Fockens P, Dekker E (2014) Random biopsies taken during colonoscopic surveillance of patients with longstanding ulcerative colitis: low yield and absence of clinical consequences. Am J Gastroenterol 109(5):715–722, doi:ajg201193 [pii] 10.1038/ajg.2011.93
107. Kiesslich R, Fritsch J, Holtmann M, Koehler HH, Stolte M, Kanzler S, Nafe B, Jung M, Galle PR, Neurath MF (2003) Methylene blue-aided chromoendoscopy for the detection of intraepithelial neoplasia and colon cancer in ulcerative colitis. Gastroenterology 124 (4):880–888, doi:10.1053/gast.2003.50146 S001650850300060X [pii]
108. Fujii S, Fujimori T, Chiba T (2003) Usefulness of analysis of p53 alteration and observation of surface microstructure for diagnosis of ulcerative colitis-associated colorectal neoplasia. J Exp Clin Cancer Res 22(1):107–115

109. Toyota M, Ahuja N, Ohe-Toyota M, Herman JG, Baylin SB, Issa JP (1999) CpG island methylator phenotype in colorectal cancer. Proc Natl Acad Sci U S A 96(15):8681–8686
110. Issa JP, Ottaviano YL, Celano P, Hamilton SR, Davidson NE, Baylin SB (1994) Methylation of the oestrogen receptor CpG island links ageing and neoplasia in human colon. Nat Genet 7 (4):536–540. doi:10.1038/ng0894-536
111. Fujii S, Tominaga K, Kitajima K, Takeda J, Kusaka T, Fujita M, Ichikawa K, Tomita S, Ohkura Y, Ono Y, Imura J, Chiba T, Fujimori T (2005) Methylation of the oestrogen receptor gene in non-neoplastic epithelium as a marker of colorectal neoplasia risk in longstanding and extensive ulcerative colitis. Gut 54(9):1287–1292, doi:gut.2004.062059 [pii] 10.1136/gut.2004.062059
112. Tominaga K, Fujii S, Mukawa K, Fujita M, Ichikawa K, Tomita S, Imai Y, Kanke K, Ono Y, Terano A, Hiraishi H, Fujimori T (2005) Prediction of colorectal neoplasia by quantitative methylation analysis of estrogen receptor gene in nonneoplastic epithelium from patients with ulcerative colitis. Clin Cancer Res 11(24 Pt 1):8880–8885, doi:11/24/8880 [pii] 10.1158/1078-0432.CCR-05-1309
113. Deng G, Kakar S, Kim YS (2011) MicroRNA-124a and microRNA-34b/c are frequently methylated in all histological types of colorectal cancer and polyps, and in the adjacent normal mucosa. Oncol Lett 2(1):175–180, doi:10.3892/ol.2010.222 ol-02-01-0175 [pii]
114. Balaguer F, Link A, Lozano JJ, Cuatrecasas M, Nagasaka T, Boland CR, Goel A (2010) Epigenetic silencing of miR-137 is an early event in colorectal carcinogenesis. Cancer Res 70 (16):6609–6618, doi:0008-5472.CAN-10-0622 [pii] 10.1158/0008-5472.CAN-10-0622
115. Lujambio A, Ropero S, Ballestar E, Fraga MF, Cerrato C, Setien F, Casado S, Suarez-Gauthier A, Sanchez-Cespedes M, Git A, Spiteri I, Das PP, Caldas C, Miska E, Esteller M (2007) Genetic unmasking of an epigenetically silenced microRNA in human cancer cells. Cancer Res 67(4):1424–1429, doi:67/4/1424 [pii] 10.1158/0008-5472.CAN-06-4218
116. Hudson RS, Yi M, Esposito D, Watkins SK, Hurwitz AA, Yfantis HG, Lee DH, Borin JF, Naslund MJ, Alexander RB, Dorsey TH, Stephens RM, Croce CM, Ambs S (2012) MicroRNA-1 is a candidate tumor suppressor and prognostic marker in human prostate cancer. Nucleic Acids Res 40(8):3689–3703, doi:gkr1222 [pii] 10.1093/nar/gkr1222
117. Yu T, Liu K, Wu Y, Fan J, Chen J, Li C, Yang Q, Wang Z (2013) MicroRNA-9 inhibits the proliferation of oral squamous cell carcinoma cells by suppressing expression of CXCR4 via the Wnt/beta-catenin signaling pathway. Oncogene. doi:onc2013448 [pii] 10.1038/onc.2013.448
118. Toiyama Y, Hur K, Tanaka K, Inoue Y, Tabata T, Kusunoki M, Boland CR, Goel A (2013) Methylated miR-124, -137, and -34b/c as predictive biomarkers for ulcerative colitis-associated colorectal neoplasia. J Clin Oncol 31:(suppl; abstr e14631)

Part III
Surgical Treatment

Chapter 6
Surgical Treatment for Ulcerative Colitis-Associated Cancer or Dysplasia

Toshimitsu Araki, Yuji Toiyama, Yoshiki Okita, Koji Tanaka, Yasuhiro Inoue, Keiichi Uchida, and Masato Kusunoki

Abstract Patients with long-standing ulcerative colitis (UC) have an increased risk of colorectal neoplasia (from dysplasia to advanced cancer) and are therefore candidates for several kinds of surgical treatments, ranging from an endoscopic resection to abdominoperineal resection and total proctocolectomy, depending on disease status. In addition to the extent of resection, patient age and sex, anal function, UC status, and type or location of the neoplasia must be taken into account in surgical decision-making. Although total proctocolectomy with ileal pouch-anal anastomosis is the gold standard for UC-associated colorectal cancer, the pros and cons of rectal mucosectomy are still debated. In addition, the postoperative administration of immunomodulators or biologics for UC is controversial. Data on the prognosis of surgically treated patients are still limited, and conclusions cannot yet be drawn. However, these patients should be closely followed for a relapse of inflammation and the recurrence of neoplasia in the residual lesion, especially in the anal transition zone. Recent, more aggressive approaches include chemoradiotherapy followed by ileal pouch-anal anastomosis or partial intersphincteric resection.

Keywords Ulcerative colitis • Surgery • Colorectal cancer • Dysplasia • Ileal pouch

6.1 Introduction

Previously, 25 % of the patients with ulcerative colitis (UC) underwent colectomy for medically refractory UC or UC-associated neoplasia. In recent years, however, elective colectomy rates in UC patients have decreased, as the efficacy of antitumor necrosis factor (TNF) antibodies has been confirmed and their use has increased significantly [1]. Nonetheless, patients with long-standing UC continue to be at

T. Araki (✉) • Y. Toiyama • Y. Okita • K. Tanaka • Y. Inoue • K. Uchida • M. Kusunoki
Department of Gastrointestinal and Pediatric Surgery, Division of Reparative Medicine, Institute of Life Sciences, Mie University Graduate School of Medicine, 2-174 Edobashi, Tsu, Mie 514-8507, Japan
e-mail: taraki@clin.medic.mie-u.ac.jp

M. Kusunoki (ed.), *Colitis-Associated Cancer*, DOI 10.1007/978-4-431-55522-3_6

higher risk of colorectal cancer (CRC) than the general population and therefore often require surgery for UC-associated neoplasia. The early detection of cancers in UC patients means that the tumor can be treated at an earlier stage, which corresponds to a better prognosis [2].

Total proctocolectomy (PC) with ileal pouch-anal anastomosis (IPAA) is the procedure of choice for patients undergoing elective surgery for UC and is the standard procedure for those with UC-associated CRC. Clearly, there are fewer indications for IPAA in the treatment of UC-associated neoplasia than for medically refractory UC, given that in the treatment of CRC, the primary aim is to improve the oncologic prognosis, which takes precedence over the functional prognosis.

Recent technical progress in gastroenterological endoscopy has allowed the more accurate detection of dysplasia, which has led to renewed debate regarding the utility of endoscopic surveillance or resection for dysplastic lesions. The larger proportion of younger patients with UC-associated cancer than sporadic cancer in individuals with a normal mucosa has also led to a reconsideration of surgery for UC-associated cancer with respect to operative indication, extent of resection, and pros and cons of rectal mucosectomy. In this chapter, we discuss the various options for the surgical treatment of UC-associated cancer while taking into account the related controversies.

6.2 Surgical Indications for UC-Associated Neoplasia

Although the choice of treatment is influenced by the site and stage of the cancer, the detection of CRC by biopsy is an absolute indication for surgery in UC patients. UC-associated cancer is characterized by its broad range of macroscopic appearances, its tendency to spread diffusely and invasively, and its poorly marginated lesions; these features distinguish it from sporadic CRC [3]. Another important difference between sporadic and UC-related colonic neoplasia is that in the latter the entire colonic mucosa is at risk for neoplastic transformation, which can be multifocal [4]. The underlying mechanism is the inflammation → dysplasia → carcinoma sequence in patients with long-standing UC-related inflammation of the colon and rectum [5–7]. In addition, so-called field effects of multiple epigenetic alterations, including methylation, have been shown in both the neoplastic and non-dysplastic mucosa of UC patients [8–10]. Field effects have been attributed to the constant reepithelialization of the ulcerated and chronically inflamed colonic mucosa by abnormal cell clones that arise during healing and subsequently expand [11] and to changes in the local environment, such as oxidative stress and an altered bacterial flora, both of which can give rise to cellular mutations [12].

Dysplasia, the earliest histologic manifestation of neoplastic transformation, is defined as an unequivocal neoplastic change in the colonic epithelium without invasion into the lamina propria. Dysplasia is grouped into five main categories: low-grade dysplasia (LGD), high-grade dysplasia (HGD), dysplasia-associated lesion or mass (DALM), adenoma-like mass (ALM), and adenoma-like DALM. The appearance of any of these is an early clinical alert to the development of carcinogenesis because the probability of a coexistent carcinoma is relatively high [13, 14]. However, some researchers maintain that the presence of dysplasia is associated with a low risk of unsuspected cancer at the time of colectomy [15]. Accordingly, the decision-making process for patients with UC who are considering intensive surveillance vs. surgical intervention after a diagnosis of dysplasia is a controversial one.

6.2.1 High-Grade Dysplasia

Over 30 % of the patients with HGD will develop cancer during subsequent surveillances; however, there are no reported instances in which HGD was subsequently downgraded to negative [7, 16, 17]. Among patients with HGD who underwent prophylactic colectomy immediately after diagnosis, about 40 % had cancer in the resected sample [7, 18–20]. Moreover, the HGD was detected at a colonic site distant from that of the synchronously detected cancer [19, 21]. Therefore, a diagnosis of HGD is an absolute indication for surgical resection [22–24].

6.2.2 Low-Grade Dysplasia

Whether patients with flat LGD should undergo surgery continues to be debated. Among patients with LGD with subsequent surveillance colonoscopy, 5–50 % subsequently had the diagnosis downgraded to indefinite or negative [17, 18, 20, 25]. However, in approximately 30 % of these patients, there was eventual progression to HGD, DALM, or cancer [7, 16–18, 20, 22, 25]. Cancer was eventually detected in approximately 10 % of the patients with LGD and subsequent surveillances [16, 18, 20, 22, 25–27]. Zisman et al. [28] showed that patients with three or more biopsies demonstrating LGD at a single colonoscopy had an increased risk of progression to advanced neoplasia [relative risk (RR) = 5.8; 95 % confidence interval (CI): 1.29–26.04].

Analyses of the outcomes of patients who underwent colonoscopic surveillance for 10 years following the detection of LGD did not show a statistically significant difference from the outcomes of control patients. This conclusion is supported by histopathologic reviews, which have demonstrated the unreliability of LGD diagnosis [29]. Thus, the current opinion is that a diagnosis of LGD does not justify prophylactic colectomy.

However, there are opposing views regarding whether only flat lesions should be followed up endoscopically, because dysplastic lesions, which eventually progress to invasive cancer, cannot be consistently and reliably detected through successive surveillances [30]. Bernstein et al. [22] analyzed ten prospective studies (1225 patients), in which the lesions of 16–29 % of the patients progressed from untreated LGD to DALM, HGD, or cancer. In their retrospective study, Kiran et al. [31] showed that the rate of the risk of cancer in postoperative pathologic findings was 3 % even if preoperative biopsies demonstrated LGD. In general, because advanced neoplasia can be found in association with dysplastic changes of any grade, patients with confirmed dysplasia of any grade should undergo colectomy [13, 22, 26, 31, 32].

According to the current American College of Gastroenterology guideline [33], surgery should be promptly considered in patients with flat LGD to prevent progression to a higher grade of neoplasia. In the Medical Position Statement of the American Gastroenterological Association [34, 35], multifocal LGD is a strong indication for colectomy. In addition, although controversial, there is evidence to suggest that patients with flat, unifocal, LGD should also be considered for colectomy [36, 37].

Primary sclerosing cholangitis (PSC) is typically associated with inflammatory bowel disease (IBD), particularly UC. PSC-IBD patients are at an increased risk of colorectal neoplasia [38]. In one-third of PSC-UC patients, LGD will progress to HGD/CRC. Venkatesh et al. [39] evaluated ten PSC-UC patients with LGD who underwent surveillance colonoscopy. In three (30 %) patients, LGD progressed to raised HGD over a mean follow-up of 13 ± 11 months, and HGD occurred more frequently within the first year of the initial detection of LGD (23.5 per 100 patient-years of follow-up). Therefore, PSC-UC patients with LGD should be closely and carefully followed.

6.2.3 Dysplasia-Associated Lesion or Mass

It was initially suggested that any dysplasia found in association with a DALM, in particular with a polypoid mass, indicates a high likelihood of the presence of synchronous or metachronous neoplasia [40]. Bernstein et al. [22] evaluated 40 patients with DALM from ten prospective studies (1225 patients); 17 (43 %) of the patients already had cancer at immediate colectomy. In another report of patients with HGD in DALM who were followed for over 5 years, none of the patients had carcinoma, either in surveillance biopsies or in resection specimens [41]. Thus, the latter authors concluded that the presence of HGD in DALMs does not warrant colectomy with continued close observation.

In a series of 348 patients from 1984 to 2007, Kiran et al. [31] demonstrated that those with a preoperatively detected DALM had a significantly higher risk of cancer than patients with flat dysplasia (25 % vs. 8 %; $P < 0.001$). They also found that the risk of cancer was not significantly higher in LGD with DALM than in flat LGD (7 % vs. 2 %; $P = 0.3$), but the risk of cancer or HGD was threefold higher (29 % vs. 9 %; $P = 0.015$).

Recent studies broadly separated the raised (endoscopically visible) dysplastic lesions in IBD into those resembling non-IBD-related sporadic adenomas (adenoma-like) and those that do not resemble adenomas (non-adenoma-like) [42–44]. Biopsy specimens of non-adenoma-like DALMs may contain the surface of an invasive adenocarcinoma, which is regarded as endoscopically unresectable [40]. Thus, patients with UC and an endoscopically unresectable, non-adenoma-like DALM, regardless of the grade of dysplasia detected on biopsy analysis, should undergo colectomy, because of the high association of these lesions with metachronous or synchronous carcinoma [35, 45].

6.2.4 Stricture

A colonic stricture is regarded as a manifestation of chronic UC, although carcinoma may occur at the site of a stricture [46], and a fibrous stricture as an indication for surgery, owing to the possibility of malignant degeneration [47]. Gumaste et al. [14] investigated 1156 UC patients; in this group, 17 of the 70 strictures (24 %) proved to harbor a malignancy. In addition, they described three features that distinguish a malignant from a benign stricture: (1) appearance late in the course of UC (61 % probability of malignancy in strictures that develop after 20 years of disease vs. 0 % in those occurring before 10 years); (2) location proximal to the splenic flexure (86 % vs. 47 %, 10 %, and 0 % when the stricture is in the sigmoid colon, rectum, and splenic flexure and descending colon, respectively); and (3) symptomatic large bowel obstruction (100 % probability of malignancy vs. 14 % in the absence of obstruction or constipation) [14]. Lashner et al. [48] described 15 patients with UC-related strictures identified by air-contrast barium enema or on colonoscopy; within this group, 11 had dysplasia and two had cancer. Thus, a stricture should be considered as a strong risk factor for cancer, requiring intensive colonoscopic surveillance. If dysplasia is discovered or if the stricture cannot be adequately biopsied, then surgical treatment should be considered [48].

6.3 Surgical Procedure

The surgical procedure for neoplasia in patients with UC varies, ranging from colonoscopic resection to total PC. Although PC with permanent ileostomy and restorative PC with mucosectomy are the only surgical procedures that will reliably eliminate the cancer risk in UC, the risk of subsequent morbidity and impaired anal function is not small. The choice of surgical treatment is influenced by the site and stage of the neoplasia, the functional state of the rectum, the presence of multifocal lesions, the patient's age, and the duration of UC [49] (Fig. 6.1).

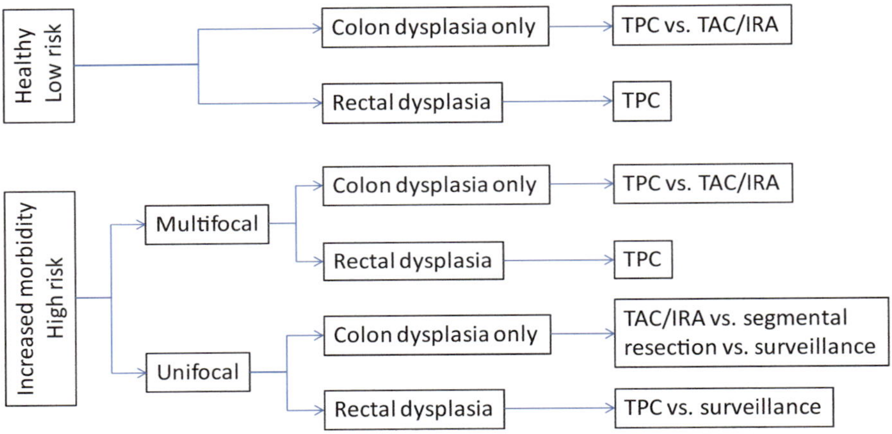

Fig. 6.1 Surgical options for ulcerative colitis patients with dysplasia found on colonoscopy. *IPAA* ileal pouch-anal anastomosis, *IRA* ileorectal anastomosis, *TAC* total abdominal colectomy, *TPC* total proctocolectomy

6.3.1 Abdominoperineal Total PC

Abdominoperineal total PC is the most definitive treatment for the eradication of undiagnosed synchronous dysplasias and/or carcinomas and the prevention of subsequent metachronous lesions in UC. It allows the resection of synchronous colonic and rectal dysplasia/cancer and avoids the development of metachronous colonic and rectal lesions. It also obviates the need for further colonoscopic surveillance. However, patients must accept a permanent stoma and the postoperative complications are significant, including urinary and sexual dysfunction or a nonhealing perineal wound.

Although this procedure is not an attractive option for patients with comorbidities or for those wanting to preserve anal function, it is indicated for patients with advanced rectal and anal canal cancer or for patients with poor anal sphincter function, such as the older postpartum female. These patients will also require an end ileostomy or a continent Kock ileal pouch.

6.3.2 Segmental/Partial Resection

There is limited debate regarding segmental colectomy in the treatment of lesions in patients with UC in long-standing remission. The indication for the procedures considers the difficulty of further PC and IPAA after lymphadenectomy or adhesions at the target surgical site.

Segmental colectomy is a short operative procedure and maintains continence, but most patients will later require not only further medication but also excision and colectomy and ileostomy. Moreover, a right-sided colo-anal anastomosis is unsuitable for the treatment of left-sided UC [50]. Thus, in general, partial resection of the colon should be avoided because of the high frequency of occult carcinomas and multifocal carcinogenesis. Schwarz et al. [51] reported the case of a patient who underwent a left hemicolectomy and a mucosal proctectomy but then had a macroscopic recurrence of the colitis within 2 months postoperatively and eventually required excision of the remaining colon and an end ileostomy. This suggests that the risk of UC relapse in the residual colon must be taken into account, even if the right side of the colon seems to be in remission.

Patients with UC-associated CRC have a twofold higher mortality than patients with sporadic CRC [52]. Whether segmental or partial resection is the optimal procedure for UC patients with sporadic cancer remains questionable.

6.3.3 Total Abdominal Colectomy with Ileorectal Anastomosis

The cumulative probability of total abdominal colectomy with ileorectal anastomosis (IRA) after 10 years of UC is about 50 %. Total excision was performed following the detection of dysplasia in 5.9 % of these patients [53] and is no longer an acceptable procedure for patients with UC. Although UC is generally considered to always involve the rectum and in some patients also the more proximal portions of the colon, albeit in a diffuse and non-segmental fashion, rectal sparing has been documented [53–57]. If the colitis is totally quiescent or shows rectal sparing, total abdominal colectomy with IRA may be an option for UC patients with a single cancer in the colon. However, since most colectomy specimens with an absence of macroscopic activity show histologic features of chronicity or activity [58], these patients should be monitored for a relapse of proctitis.

The indication of low anterior resection for patients with quiescent UC and rectal cancer or dysplasia should be considered very carefully, because further PC and IPAA would be difficult after this procedure. In addition, patients undergoing total abdominal colectomy with IRA and treated postoperatively with immunomodulators or biologics have a risk of a relapse of inflammation in the residual rectum. Thus, the prognosis, and especially the risk of cancer in the residual rectum, after IRA in patients with UC-associated cancer is a concern. Among patients who received an IRA, regardless of the indication, the estimated cumulative cancer risk after a disease duration of 20 years is 2.1–20.0 % [59–63]. The high long-term risk of cancer after total abdominal colectomy with IRA suggests that this procedure is an interim solution in younger patients. However, IRA with a close follow-up still plays a major role in treating UC patients because it is an easier surgical procedure than IPAA, has excellent functional results, shorter hospitalization, and, importantly, fewer severe complications, unlike in IRA [61].

A particular indication of IRA for UC-associated cancer is a non-obstructing tumor located above the pelvic floor with remote metastases in remission. In the case of an advanced tumor causing obstruction, then a primary colectomy and IRA with a covering ileostomy is advisable.

6.3.4 Subtotal Colectomy

Subtotal colectomy (STC) with end ileostomy and rectal stump pouch are less ideal options because of the retained rectum, which poses a continued cancer risk. However, STC was shown to be a safe treatment option for patients satisfied with an ileostomy or for those with comorbidities that make them ineligible for other procedures or who do not choose to undergo later pelvic pouch surgery. Nonetheless, the potential for the proliferation of residual dysplastic cells or malignant change within the rectal stump in patients who have undergone STC with rectal stump preservation for UC-associated CRC is of serious concern. In addition, whether the potential for malignancy in the rectal stump of STC patients with UC-associated CRC outweighs the morbidity associated with complete proctectomy is difficult to determine. The rate of cancer occurrence later on was shown to be low (1.4 %) in one study [62] but eightfold higher in another [64]. PSC and disease duration until STC were shown to be significant risk factors for rectal stump cancer in a closed rectal stump after STC [65]. Thus, considering the risk of rectal cancer, the low success rate of long-term rectal preservation, and the safety of surgery, a more aggressive approach to early complete proctectomy is recommended in this situation. If this is not possible, patients treated with STC should be followed with close endoscopic surveillance of the closed rectal stump.

6.3.5 Total Proctocolectomy with IPAA

IPAA by ileal J pouch, first described in 1980, is now the gold standard surgical procedure for UC refractory to medical treatment [66]. The long-term quality of life of these patients after this procedure is excellent and the level of fecal continence is satisfactory [67–69]. However, this procedure also has several technical difficulties such as mesenteric lengthening of the pouch [70, 71] and mucosal proctectomy [72]. For surgeons, extensive experience is required to obtain acceptable results [73]. Patients with refractory UC who suffer complications after PC have a poor quality of life [74]. Thus, a double-stapled anastomosis without mucosal proctectomy is the preferred procedure, as there are fewer anastomotic complications and superior rectal continence is achieved; however, a cuff of rectal mucosa is retained, which is the main concern as well as the main argument of opponents of the double-stapling technique. Whether with or without mucosal proctectomy, IPAA is indicated for any colonic or rectal lesion in the surgically fit patient who has unifocal or multifocal dysplasia and refuses a stoma. Relative contraindications of IPAA for UC-associated neoplasias are preoperative incontinence/poor anal sphincter tonus, severe backwash ileitis suggesting Crohn's disease, and very low rectal or anal dysplasia that threatens the sphincters.

However, the use of a stapled anastomosis without mucosal proctectomy in patients with UC-related dysplasia or cancer remains controversial because of the risk of developing synchronous or metachronous neoplasias in the retained anal transitional zone (ATZ) mucosa. Although an association has yet to be reported between dysplasia and any the following: age, sex, preoperative length of disease, use of a double- vs. single-staple technique, or anastomotic distance from the dentate line [75], the risk of cancer can be reduced by ensuring that the minimal length of rectal columnar mucosa is retained. It is therefore recommended that, in carrying out a stapled IPAA, the anastomosis is performed at the anorectal junction, about 1–1.5 cm above the dentate line, because of the deterioration in anorectal function [76]. Additionally, this procedure is indicated for patients with UC and right-sided colon cancers who require lymph node dissection along the superior mesenteric vein and excision of the marginal arcade of the ileocolic artery, because an insufficient extension of the ileal pouch to the anus precludes a hand-sewn IPAA with mucosectomy.

Stapled IPAA has also been advocated in patients with UC associated with coexisting neoplasia [77, 78]. In these cases, long-term surveillance to monitor dysplasia is recommended; if repeat biopsy confirms persistent dysplasia, ATZ excision with a neoileal pouch-anal anastomosis should be performed [78]. However, restorative PC with mucosectomy does not necessarily eliminate the risks, as after this procedure cancer can occur in a residual ATZ [79, 80]. Thus, in patients with long-standing ileal pouches even after mucosectomy of ATZ, and especially in cases in which dysplasia or cancer is detected in the PC specimen, routine long-term endoscopic surveillance is recommended.

There are many reported cases in the indexed medical literature of carcinoma arising after stapled IPAA for UC [79]. In some studies, the incidence of dysplasia in the ATZ at the time of total colectomy was 2.5–5 %, and duration of UC and patient age at colectomy were significant risk factors [81, 82]. In these cases, mucosal proctectomy is the definitive procedure for patients with preoperatively detected dysplasia in the ATZ.

The incidence of dysplasia after stapled IPAA is 3.0–4.5 % [75, 76, 83]. The development of cancer in the ATZ after stapled IPAA without mucosectomy has been reported [76, 84, 85] and was shown to be significantly associated with a preoperative pathologic diagnosis of UC with concurrent dysplasia or cancer [75]. Based on these data, mucosal proctectomy and hand-sewn IPAA are strongly recommended for patients with neoplasia, especially those with cancer or HGD outside the ATZ [75, 86].

For the reasons stated above, in young patients with UC-associated cancer, mucosal proctectomy with IPAA is recommended, whereas for older patients, particularly those with lower rectal cancer who will accept a permanent stoma, total PC may be proposed. Patients older than 50 years have a significantly higher rate of concurrent dysplasia and malignant degeneration than younger patients, probably because of a longer duration of disease [87]. In these cases, restorative PC with mucosal proctectomy may reduce this risk by eliminating all of the colorectal mucosa.

Branco et al. [88] reported a case in which adenocarcinoma arose in an ileal pouch after IPAA with mucosal proctectomy performed using a cavitron ultrasonic surgical aspirator (Excel, Covidien, Boulder, CO) for UC. This method was introduced to simplify and optimize IPAA with mucosectomy and has been shown to shorten the operative time and reduce blood loss [89]. Its use, however, may increase the number of pathology specimens made uninterpretable on account of tissue ablation. Another ultrasonically activated scalpel (Harmonic; Ethicon Endo Surgery, Johnson & Johnson Medical SPA, Somerville, NJ) also shortened the operative time, decreased blood loss, and was shown to be useful for restorative PC [72]. There has been no report of adenocarcinoma arising in an ileal pouch after mucosectomy performed using this device.

6.3.6 Endoscopic Resection

The ALMs seen in UC patients are similar to those observed in non-UC patients that have been treated by standard polypectomy. This method is associated with little risk of subsequent malignancy on follow-up [42, 44, 90, 91].

An accurate pathologic diagnosis is very important for distinguishing among the different pathologic entities, given the different therapeutic consequences, such as endoscopic polypectomy for ALM and potential PC for DALM. New and emerging endoscopic imaging techniques, such as chromoendoscopy, magnification endoscopy, and confocal laser endomicroscopy, provide a more accurate diagnosis. Endoscopic resection of an ALM allows confirmation of the biopsy-based adenoma diagnosis and the exclusion of a DALM [91]. However, the endoscopic resectability of a lesion is more important than whether it is an ALM or a DALM [92]. The basic rules for the detection of neoplasia [93] (Table 6.1) should be taken into account and applied in accordance with international guidelines [95–97].

Only a few studies have examined the clinical outcomes of DALMs resembling ALMs that are removed with endoscopic polypectomy, but the safety and efficacy of endoscopic resection have been evaluated [93, 94, 98]. Since DALMs, in particular those with a polypoid mass, are an indicator of a high likelihood of the presence of synchronous or metachronous neoplasia, endoscopic resection is not appropriate [22, 40].

Table 6.1 Basic rules for detecting neoplasia in patients with UC

1. Consult with experienced gastroenterologist
2. Endoscopic and bioptic control in remission phase
3. Examination outside routine schedule without time limitation
4. Ileocolonoscopy with special focus on the detection of DALMs and step (quadrant) biopsies from the rectum to the cecum in 10-cm intervals (sigmoid and rectum: quadrant biopsies at 5-cm intervals)
5. ALMs with low-grade intraepithelial neoplasia and clear-cut margins can be resected endoscopically
6. Consult with experienced histopathologist who has all clinical and endoscopy data readily available
7. Second opinion recommended in cases of histological diagnosis of neoplasia

From [94]

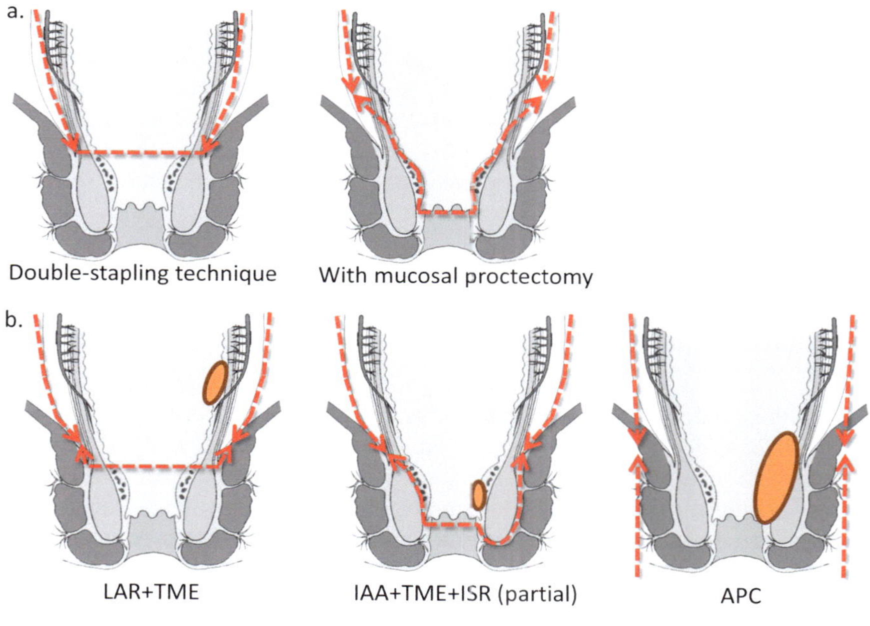

Fig. 6.2 Perianal resection line. Ileal pouch-anal anastomosis (IPAA) for ulcerative colitis (UC) (**a**), UC-associated low rectal neoplasia (**b**). *TME* total mesorectal excision, *LAR* low anterior resection, *IAA* ileoanal anastomosis, *ISR* intersphincteric resection, *APC* abdominoperineal total proctocolectomy

6.3.7 Perianal Resection Line for Rectal and Anal Canal Neoplasia

In an IPAA performed in a patient with UC without colorectal neoplasia (Fig. 6.2a.), the mesorectum is resected on the inside, close to the rectal wall, to preserve autonomic nerve function. In patients with UC-associated low rectal

Table 6.2 Indication and procedure for mesorectal excision in UC patients with rectal and anal canal cancer

Tumor status	Procedure
T1	IPAA with mucosal proctectomy (TME is recommended, taking into consideration the risk of a deeper level of T2)
Deeper level of T2 and not lower than 4 cm from the anal verge	IPAA with mucosal proctectomy and TME
Deeper level of T2 and lower than 4 cm from the anal verge	IPAA with mucosal proctectomy and TME $\pm$ ISR or APC
Deeper level of T3 or positive for lymph node metastasis	Consider preoperative chemoradiotherapy followed by APC with TME

IPAA ileal pouch-anal anastomosis, *TME* total mesorectal excision, *ISR* intersphincteric resection, *APC* abdominoperineal total proctocolectomy

neoplasia, total mesorectal excision is required in performing an IPAA (Fig. 6.2b). The choice of operative procedure depends on the depth of the tumor and its distance from the anal verge (Table 6.2). Regarding IPAA with intersphincteric resection, there are no data on postoperative anal function from a large number of cases. Thus, consensus on this procedure is lacking. Depending on curability, however, it should at most be confined to a partial intersphincteric resection (Fig. 6.2b).

6.4 Immunomodulators

Medical therapy for UC has advanced dramatically in the last decade, which has led to discussions of the pros and cons of immunomodulators or biologics for UC patients with malignant disease. Previous studies and guidelines showed that patients administered immunomodulators or biologics do not have a higher risk of new cancer development [99]. Anti-TNF antibodies have been linked to a risk of cancer recurrence in rheumatoid patients, thiopurine to a risk of cancer recurrence in transplant patients, and calcineurin inhibitor to a risk of hepatocellular carcinoma recurrence in liver transplant patients [100–102]. However, a meta-analysis of 74 random controlled trials found that anti-TNF therapies are not related to the short-term clinical emergence of cancer [103]. Nonetheless, a relapse residual lesion is not a rare occurrence after segmental/partial resection; thus, in these patients with advanced cancer, the restricted use of immunomodulators or biologics should be considered.

6.5 Prognosis

6.5.1 Neoplasia in an Ileal Pouch

Previously, cancer of the ileal mucosa was reported in patients who underwent a Brooke ileostomy [104–107] and in those with a Kock pouch [108], but the natural history and prognosis of pouch dysplasia or cancer are poorly understood. Although inflammation, villous atrophy, and colonic metaplasia have been observed within the mucosa of ileal pouches after IPAA, dysplasia may also develop, but the incidence is <0.02 % 20 years after IPAA [109].

In their study of pouch-related adenocarcinoma, Selvaggi et al. [64] showed a pooled cumulative incidence of 0.33 % 50 years after the diagnosis and 0.35 % 20 years after IPAA in a systematic review of the meta-analyses of the literature of pouch-related adenocarcinoma in patients with an IPAA for UC. In that study, one-third of the adenocarcinomas arose from the pouch as a whole and the remainder from the anorectal mucosa [64].

Derikx et al. [110] used the National Registry from 1991 to 2012 to identify 1200 patients with IBD and IPAA; 25 (1.83 %) developed pouch neoplasia, including 16 adenocarcinomas. The cumulative incidence of pouch neoplasia at 5, 10, 15, and 20 years was 1.0 %, 2.0 %, 3.7 %, and 6.9 % for pouch neoplasia and 0.6 %, 1.4 %, 2.1 %, and 3.3 % for pouch carcinoma [110] (Fig. 6.3). A history of colorectal neoplasia was the only risk factor associated with pouch neoplasia. Hazard ratios were 3.76 (95 % CI: 1.39–10.19) for prior dysplasia and 24.69 (95 % CI: 9.61–63.42) for prior carcinoma [110]. Another systematic review similarly concluded that neoplasia in the colectomy specimen was the strongest risk factor (odds ratio = 8.8; 95 % CI: 4.61–16.80) [64].

Malignant transformation of the ileal pouch mucosa may occur even in the absence of backwash ileitis or a previous history of cancer [111, 112], as determined in biopsies from the ileal pouch mucosa obtained at least 1 year after the newly formed pouch that was influenced by fecal flow [113]. Chronic inflammation of the ileal mucosa such as occurs with preoperative backwash ileitis and postoperative pouchitis in UC has also been linked to the sequence of malignant transformation [114–117]. An abnormal lesion of the ileal pouch mucosa was shown to have a high risk of adenocarcinoma 20 years or later after the initial IPAA [118].

PSC-IBD patients are at increased risk of colorectal neoplasia [38], but the development of pouch neoplasia in PSC-UC patients following IPAA is unclear. Imam et al. [119] conducted a retrospective chart review of 65 patients with PSC and IBD who underwent colectomy with IPAA followed by pouch surveillance between 1995 and 2012. The cumulative 5-year incidence of pouch neoplasia was 5.6 % (95 % CI, 1.8–16.1 %). Based on this short-term follow-up, they concluded that a frequent surveillance of the pouch was an unnecessary practice in PSC-IBD patients. However, it is recommended that patients with these risk factors be followed by endoscopy and random biopsies for the rest of their lives. If a pouch-

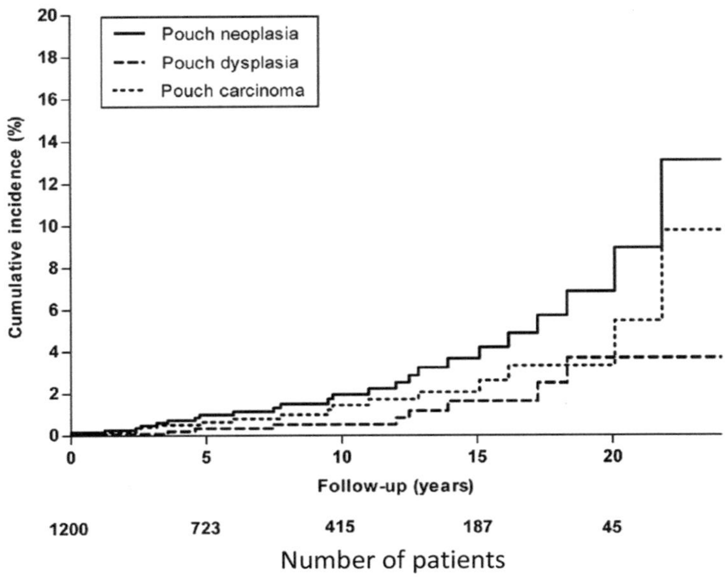

Fig. 6.3 Cumulative incidences of pouch neoplasia (both carcinoma and dysplasia), pouch carcinoma, and dysplasia (From [110])

related adenocarcinoma is detected during these examinations, abdominoperineal excision is recommended.

6.5.2 Outcome of Colorectal Cancer in UC

There have been a few reports based on small series that examined the outcome of patients with UC and CRC [12, 120–123]. From a functional aspect, among cancer patients who received an IPAA, no significant differences could be found between those with UC-associated CRC and those with UC without CRC [124]. For UC-associated CRCs, as for non-colitic cancers, histologic stage, site, and mucin content of the tumor are the most important variables determining postoperative survival [49].

A 20-year follow-up study of IBD-related CRC from the Mayo Clinic compared patients with sporadic CRC with age- and sex-matched patients with IBD-related cancers. In the latter group, the tumors were more proximally located, with only 55 % distal to the splenic flexure, compared with 78 % among patients with sporadic CRC [125]. However, compared with sporadic tumors, IBD-related CRC was more often in an advanced stage and more likely to have a mucinous component [125]. Yet, no differences were found in the overall survival of patients with sporadic CRC and those with IBD-related CRC [125].

Heimann et al. [126] showed that the 5-year survival rate was significantly worse for patients with non-diploid tumors (76 % vs. 32 %). When stratified by stage, only patients with Dukes' C lesions had a significant difference in survival for diploid vs. non-diploid tumors. Multivariate analysis showed that Dukes' classification was the best prognostic indicator, followed by tumor differentiation and DNA ploidy. Tumor location, colloid content, number of cancers, duration of disease, and patient age and sex did not correlate with the prognosis [126].

A retrospective review of 1642 UC patients by Kavanagh et al. [127] showed that patients who undergo surgery for UC-associated CRC ($n=22$) have less favorable short-term outcomes but present at a less advanced stage and have a more favorable long-term prognosis than similar patients with CRC and Crohn's disease. The overall 5-year survival was significantly better in the UC group than in the group with Crohn's disease (41 % vs. 29 %; $P=0.04$).

Watanabe et al. [128] showed that in a group of 108,536 CRC patients, the 169 with UC-associated CRC had a poorer survival than patients with sporadic CRC (43.3 % vs. 57.4 %; $P=0.0320$) for stage III disease but not for early-stage disease. The authors concluded that the detection of UC-associated CRC at an early stage results in similar postoperative outcomes as those of patients with sporadic CRC. A Danish population-based study also compared patients with UC-associated CRC ($n=279$) and those with sporadic CRC ($n=71{,}259$). Cancer stage and rates of lymph node and distant metastasis were similar between the two groups, but the overall mortality rates at 1 and 5 years after cancer diagnosis were higher in UC-associated CRC than in sporadic CRC (OR = 1.24; 95 % CI: 1.02–1.51 and OR = 1.17; 95 % CI: 1.01–1.36, respectively) [129]. Other population-based studies showed that patients diagnosed with UC-associated CRC at age <60 years had a worse outcome [130, 131], which, according to Shu et al. [131], was more pronounced in males.

6.5.3 *Radiation/Chemotherapy*

Although locally advanced rectal cancer requiring multimodality therapy is uncommon in patients with UC, the functional outcome of patients with UC-associated CRC who received adjuvant chemotherapy was shown to be very good if the appropriate surgical technique and chemotherapy protocol were selected [86].

Preoperative chemoradiotherapy (CRT) and total mesorectal excision with or without intersphincteric excision are the current treatment choices for patients with lower rectal cancer. This approach was shown to optimize oncologic outcome and to maintain anorectal function [132]. By contrast, pelvic radiation administered prior to IPAA is associated with poor pouch outcomes for UC patients [86, 133, 134]. In fact, external beam radiation to treat cancer is problematic in UC patients, especially because the small bowel has a lower tolerance than the large bowel [135]. Thus, whether adjuvant CRT increases postoperative complications remains controversial [133, 136].

In patients with cancer located in the ATZ and close to the internal sphincter, restorative PC and partial intersphincteric resection may be indicated [136], whereas preoperative CRT has a negative impact on sphincter function [136–138]. A recent report identified preoperative CRT as a risk factor for impaired anal function after intersphincteric resection [139]. CRT followed by IPAA and partial intersphincteric resection may be even more destructive in terms of postoperative anal function, with several studies showing better outcomes than colonic J pouch reconstruction for lower rectal cancer [140–142]. Previous reports demonstrated a high tolerance of preoperative CRT and pouch surgery with minimum intersphincteric resection [142, 143]. Overall, because prognosis seems to be related to cancer stage, the oncologic benefits and pouch functional outcomes should be carefully balanced before pelvic radiation prior to IPAA is considered [134].

References

1. Kaplan GG et al (2012) Decreasing colectomy rates for ulcerative colitis: a population-based time trend study. Am J Gastroenterol 107(12):1879–1887
2. Mpofu C, Watson AJ, Rhodes JM (2004) Strategies for detecting colon cancer and/or dysplasia in patients with inflammatory bowel disease. Cochrane Database Syst Rev 2: CD000279
3. Eaden JA, Abrams KR, Mayberry JF (2001) The risk of colorectal cancer in ulcerative colitis: a meta-analysis. Gut 48(4):526–535
4. Ullman TA, Itzkowitz SH (2011) Intestinal inflammation and cancer. Gastroenterology 140 (6):1807–1816
5. Riddell RH et al (1983) Dysplasia in inflammatory bowel disease: standardized classification with provisional clinical applications. Hum Pathol 14(11):931–968
6. Melville DM et al (1988) Dysplasia and deoxyribonucleic acid aneuploidy in the assessment of precancerous changes in chronic ulcerative colitis. Observer variation and correlations. Gastroenterology 95(3):668–675
7. Lofberg R et al (1990) Colonoscopic surveillance in long-standing total ulcerative colitis–a 15-year follow-up study. Gastroenterology 99(4):1021–1031
8. Burmer GC et al (1992) Neoplastic progression in ulcerative colitis: histology, DNA content, and loss of a p53 allele. Gastroenterology 103(5):1602–1610
9. Leedham SJ et al (2009) Clonality, founder mutations, and field cancerization in human ulcerative colitis-associated neoplasia. Gastroenterology 136(2):542–550, e6
10. Galandiuk S et al (2012) Field cancerization in the intestinal epithelium of patients with Crohn's ileocolitis. Gastroenterology 142(4):855–864, e8
11. Lyda MH et al (2000) Microsatellite instability and K-ras mutations in patients with ulcerative colitis. Hum Pathol 31(6):665–671
12. Itzkowitz SH, Yio X (2004) Inflammation and cancer IV. Colorectal cancer in inflammatory bowel disease: the role of inflammation. Am J Physiol Gastrointest Liver Physiol 287(1):G7–G17
13. Gorfine SR et al (2000) Dysplasia complicating chronic ulcerative colitis: is immediate colectomy warranted? Dis Colon Rectum 43(11):1575–1581
14. Gumaste V, Sachar DB, Greenstein AJ (1992) Benign and malignant colorectal strictures in ulcerative colitis. Gut 33(7):938–941

15. Murphy J et al (2014) Dysplasia in ulcerative colitis as a predictor of unsuspected synchronous colorectal cancer. Dis Colon Rectum 57(8):993–998
16. Lennard-Jones JE et al (1990) Precancer and cancer in extensive ulcerative colitis: findings among 401 patients over 22 years. Gut 31(7):800–806
17. Leidenius M et al (1991) Dysplasia and carcinoma in longstanding ulcerative colitis: an endoscopic and histological surveillance programme. Gut 32(12):1521–1525
18. Nugent FW, Haggitt RC, Gilpin PA (1991) Cancer surveillance in ulcerative colitis. Gastroenterology 100(5 Pt 1):1241–1248
19. Lashner BA, Kane SV, Hanauer SB (1990) Colon cancer surveillance in chronic ulcerative colitis: historical cohort study. Am J Gastroenterol 85(9):1083–1087
20. Lynch DA et al (1993) Failure of colonoscopic surveillance in ulcerative colitis. Gut 34 (8):1075–1080
21. Lashner BA, Silverstein MD, Hanauer SB (1989) Hazard rates for dysplasia and cancer in ulcerative colitis. Results from a surveillance program. Dig Dis Sci 34(10):1536–1541
22. Bernstein CN, Shanahan F, Weinstein WM (1994) Are we telling patients the truth about surveillance colonoscopy in ulcerative colitis? Lancet 343(8889):71–74
23. Saito Y et al (1995) Total colectomy and ileorectal anastomosis in ulcerative colitis. J Gastroenterol 30(Suppl 8):131–134
24. Nugent FW et al (1979) Malignant potential of chronic ulcerative colitis. Preliminary report. Gastroenterology 76(1):1–5
25. Woolrich AJ, DaSilva MD, Korelitz BI (1992) Surveillance in the routine management of ulcerative colitis: the predictive value of low-grade dysplasia. Gastroenterology 103 (2):431–438
26. Ullman T et al (2003) Progression of flat low-grade dysplasia to advanced neoplasia in patients with ulcerative colitis. Gastroenterology 125(5):1311–1319
27. Connell WR et al (1994) Factors affecting the outcome of endoscopic surveillance for cancer in ulcerative colitis. Gastroenterology 107(4):934–944
28. Zisman TL et al (2012) Prospective study of the progression of low-grade dysplasia in ulcerative colitis using current cancer surveillance guidelines. Inflamm Bowel Dis 18 (12):2240–2246
29. Lim CH et al (2003) Ten year follow up of ulcerative colitis patients with and without low grade dysplasia. Gut 52(8):1127–1132
30. Itzkowitz SH, Harpaz N (2004) Diagnosis and management of dysplasia in patients with inflammatory bowel diseases. Gastroenterology 126(6):1634–1648
31. Kiran RP et al (2014) Risk and location of cancer in patients with preoperative colitis-associated dysplasia undergoing proctocolectomy. Ann Surg 259(2):302–309
32. Ullman TA et al (2002) The fate of low grade dysplasia in ulcerative colitis. Am J Gastroenterol 97(4):922–927
33. Kornbluth A, Sachar DB (2010) Ulcerative colitis practice guidelines in adults: American College of Gastroenterology, Practice Parameters Committee. Am J Gastroenterol 105 (3):501–523; quiz 524
34. Farraye FA et al (2010) AGA medical position statement on the diagnosis and management of colorectal neoplasia in inflammatory bowel disease. Gastroenterology 138(2):738–745
35. Farraye FA et al (2010) AGA technical review on the diagnosis and management of colorectal neoplasia in inflammatory bowel disease. Gastroenterology 138(2):746–774, 774 e1-4; quiz e12-3
36. Itzkowitz SH, Present DH (2005) Consensus conference: colorectal cancer screening and surveillance in inflammatory bowel disease. Inflamm Bowel Dis 11(3):314–321
37. Eaden JA, Mayberry JF (2002) Guidelines for screening and surveillance of asymptomatic colorectal cancer in patients with inflammatory bowel disease. Gut 51(Suppl 5):V10–V12
38. Das P et al (2007) Risk of dysplasia and adenocarcinoma following restorative proctocolectomy for ulcerative colitis. Color Dis 9(1):15–27

39. Venkatesh PG et al (2013) Natural history of low grade dysplasia in patients with primary sclerosing cholangitis and ulcerative colitis. J Crohns Colitis 7(12):968–973
40. Blackstone MO et al (1981) Dysplasia-associated lesion or mass (DALM) detected by colonoscopy in long-standing ulcerative colitis: an indication for colectomy. Gastroenterology 80(2):366–374
41. Blonski W et al (2008) High-grade dysplastic adenoma-like mass lesions are not an indication for colectomy in patients with ulcerative colitis. Scand J Gastroenterol 43(7):817–820
42. Odze RD et al (2004) Long-term follow-up after polypectomy treatment for adenoma-like dysplastic lesions in ulcerative colitis. Clin Gastroenterol Hepatol 2(7):534–541
43. Rubin PH et al (1999) Colonoscopic polypectomy in chronic colitis: conservative management after endoscopic resection of dysplastic polyps. Gastroenterology 117(6):1295–1300
44. Engelsgjerd M, Farraye FA, Odze RD (1999) Polypectomy may be adequate treatment for adenoma-like dysplastic lesions in chronic ulcerative colitis. Gastroenterology 117 (6):1288–1294; discussion 1488–91
45. Odze RD (1999) Adenomas and adenoma-like DALMs in chronic ulcerative colitis: a clinical, pathological, and molecular review. Am J Gastroenterol 94(7):1746–1750
46. Brooke BN (1961) Malignant change in ulcerative colitis. Dis Colon Rectum 4:393–398
47. Truelove SC, Witts LJ (1955) Cortisone in ulcerative colitis; final report on a therapeutic trial. Br Med J 2(4947):1041–1048
48. Lashner BA et al (1990) Dysplasia and cancer complicating strictures in ulcerative colitis. Dig Dis Sci 35(3):349–352
49. Sugita A et al (1993) Survival with colorectal cancer in ulcerative colitis. A study of 102 cases. Ann Surg 218(2):189–195
50. Varma JS et al (1987) Mucosal proctectomy and colo-anal anastomosis for distal ulcerative proctocolitis. Br J Surg 74(5):381–383
51. Schwarz RJ, Pezim ME (1991) Failure of right-sided coloanal anastomosis for treatment of left-sided ulcerative colitis. Report of a case. Dis Colon Rectum 34(7):618–621
52. Sebastian S et al (2014) Colorectal cancer in inflammatory bowel disease: results of the 3rd ECCO pathogenesis scientific workshop (I). J Crohns Colitis 8(1):5–18
53. Glickman JN, Odze RD (2008) Does rectal sparing ever occur in ulcerative colitis? Inflamm Bowel Dis 14(Suppl 2):S166–S167
54. Bousvaros A et al (2007) Differentiating ulcerative colitis from Crohn disease in children and young adults: report of a working group of the North American Society for Pediatric Gastroenterology, Hepatology, and Nutrition and the Crohn's and Colitis Foundation of America. J Pediatr Gastroenterol Nutr 44(5):653–674
55. Rajwal SR et al (2004) Endoscopic rectal sparing in children with untreated ulcerative colitis. J Pediatr Gastroenterol Nutr 38(1):66–69
56. Robert ME et al (2004) Patterns of inflammation in mucosal biopsies of ulcerative colitis: perceived differences in pediatric populations are limited to children younger than 10 years. Am J Surg Pathol 28(2):183–189
57. Yantiss RK, Odze RD (2007) Pitfalls in the interpretation of nonneoplastic mucosal biopsies in inflammatory bowel disease. Am J Gastroenterol 102(4):890–904
58. Joo M, Odze RD (2010) Rectal sparing and skip lesions in ulcerative colitis: a comparative study of endoscopic and histologic findings in patients who underwent proctocolectomy. Am J Surg Pathol 34(5):689–696
59. Andersson P et al (2014) Ileorectal anastomosis in comparison with ileal pouch anal anastomosis in reconstructive surgery for ulcerative colitis–a single institution experience. J Crohns Colitis 8(7):582–589
60. Johnson WR et al (1986) The outcome of patients with ulcerative colitis managed by subtotal colectomy. Surg Gynecol Obstet 162(5):421–425
61. Romano G et al (1987) Role of ileorectal anastomosis in the treatment of ulcerative colitis and familial polyposis. Ital J Surg Sci 17(2):135–140

62. Oakley JR et al (1985) The fate of the rectal stump after subtotal colectomy for ulcerative colitis. Dis Colon Rectum 28(6):394–396
63. Baker WN et al (1978) Cancer of the rectum following colectomy and ileorectal anastomosis for ulcerative colitis. Br J Surg 65(12):862–868
64. Selvaggi F et al (2014) Systematic review of cuff and pouch cancer in patients with ileal pelvic pouch for ulcerative colitis. Inflamm Bowel Dis 20(7):1296–1308
65. Lutgens MW et al (2012) Risk factors for rectal stump cancer in inflammatory bowel disease. Dis Colon Rectum 55(2):191–196
66. Utsunomiya J et al (1980) Total colectomy, mucosal proctectomy, and ileoanal anastomosis. Dis Colon Rectum 23(7):459–466
67. Kim WH et al (1999) Quality of life in Korean patients with inflammatory bowel diseases: ulcerative colitis, Crohn's disease and intestinal Behcet's disease. Int J Color Dis 14(1):52–57
68. Cheung WY et al (2000) The UK IBDQ-a British version of the inflammatory bowel disease questionnaire. development and validation. J Clin Epidemiol 53(3):297–306
69. Watanabe K et al (2006) Assessment of the Japanese Inflammatory Bowel Disease Questionnaire in patients after ileal pouch anal anastomosis for ulcerative colitis. J Gastroenterol 41(7):662–667
70. Burnstein MJ et al (1987) Technique of mesenteric lengthening in ileal reservoir-anal anastomosis. Dis Colon Rectum 30(11):863–866
71. Araki T et al (2007) An alternative conversion technique for salvaging a failed ileal J-pouch-anal anastomosis to a modified H-pouch. Dig Surg 24(5):324–327
72. Kusunoki M et al (1999) Current trends in restorative proctocolectomy: introduction of an ultrasonically activated scalpel. Dis Colon Rectum 42(10):1349–1352
73. Tekkis PP et al (2005) Evaluation of the learning curve in ileal pouch-anal anastomosis surgery. Ann Surg 241(2):262–268
74. Heuschen UA et al (2002) Outcome after septic complications in J pouch procedures. Br J Surg 89(2):194–200
75. Ziv Y et al (1994) Incidence, risk factors, and treatment of dysplasia in the anal transitional zone after ileal pouch-anal anastomosis. Dis Colon Rectum 37(12):1281–1285
76. Chia CS et al (2008) Adenocarcinoma of the anal transitional zone after double stapled ileal pouch-anal anastomosis for ulcerative colitis. Color Dis 10(6):621–623
77. Al-Sukhni W et al (2010) Oncologic outcome in patients with ulcerative colitis associated with dysplasia or cancer who underwent stapled or handsewn ileal pouch-anal anastomosis. Dis Colon Rectum 53(11):1495–1500
78. O'Riordain MG et al (2000) Incidence and natural history of dysplasia of the anal transitional zone after ileal pouch-anal anastomosis: results of a five-year to ten-year follow-up. Dis Colon Rectum 43(12):1660–1665
79. Alessandroni L et al (2012) Adenocarcinoma below stapled ileoanal anastomosis after restorative proctocolectomy for ulcerative colitis. Updat Surg 64(2):149–152
80. Pedersen ME et al (2008) Adenocarcinoma arising from the rectal stump eleven years after excision of an ileal J-pouch in a patient with ulcerative colitis: report of a case. Dis Colon Rectum 51(7):1146–1148
81. Sagayama K et al (2007) Incidence of and risk factors for dysplasia in mucosectomy area in ulcerative colitis patients undergoing restorative proctocolectomy. Int J Color Dis 22 (4):439–443
82. Tsunoda A, Talbot IC, Nicholls RJ (1990) Incidence of dysplasia in the anorectal mucosa in patients having restorative proctocolectomy. Br J Surg 77(5):506–508
83. Remzi FH et al (2003) Dysplasia of the anal transitional zone after ileal pouch-anal anastomosis: results of prospective evaluation after a minimum of ten years. Dis Colon Rectum 46(1):6–13
84. Johnston D et al (1987) Preservation of the entire anal canal in conservative proctocolectomy for ulcerative colitis: a pilot study comparing end-to-end ileo-anal anastomosis without mucosal resection with mucosal proctectomy and endo-anal anastomosis. Br J Surg 74 (10):940–944

85. Galli-Gallardo SM, Pang PK, Oguro C (1979) Renal responses of the chilean toad, Calyptocephalella caudiverbera, and the mud puppy, Necturus maculosus, to mesotocin. Gen Comp Endocrinol 37(1):134–136
86. Remzi FH, Preen M (2003) Rectal cancer and ulcerative colitis: does it change the therapeutic approach? Color Dis 5(5):483–485
87. Bauer JJ et al (1997) Restorative proctocolectomy in patients older than fifty years. Dis Colon Rectum 40(5):562–565
88. Branco BC et al (2009) Adenocarcinoma complicating restorative proctocolectomy for ulcerative colitis with mucosectomy performed by Cavitron Ultrasonic Surgical Aspirator. Color Dis 11(4):428–429
89. Heimann TM et al (1984) Mucosal proctectomy using an ultrasonic scalpel. Am J Surg 147 (6):803–806
90. Monkemuller K et al (2009) Advanced colon polypectomy. Clin Gastroenterol Hepatol 7 (6):641–652
91. Vieth M, Behrens H, Stolte M (2006) Sporadic adenoma in ulcerative colitis: endoscopic resection is an adequate treatment. Gut 55(8):1151–1155
92. Rutter MD et al (2006) Thirty-year analysis of a colonoscopic surveillance program for neoplasia in ulcerative colitis. Gastroenterology 130(4):1030–1038
93. Neumann H et al (2011) Cancer risk in IBD: how to diagnose and how to manage DALM and ALM. World J Gastroenterol 17(27):3184–3191
94. Kisiel JB et al (2012) Outcome of sporadic adenomas and adenoma-like dysplasia in patients with ulcerative colitis undergoing polypectomy. Inflamm Bowel Dis 18(2):226–235
95. American Society for Gastrointestinal Endoscopy (ASGE) (1998) The role of colonoscopy in the management of patients with inflammatory bowel disease. Gastrointest Endosc 48 (6):689–690
96. Mowat C et al (2011) Guidelines for the management of inflammatory bowel disease in adults. Gut 60(5):571–607
97. Magro F et al (2013) European consensus on the histopathology of inflammatory bowel disease. J Crohns Colitis 7(10):827–851
98. Hurlstone DP et al (2007) Endoscopic mucosal resection for flat neoplasia in chronic ulcerative colitis: can we change the endoscopic management paradigm? Gut 56(6):838–846
99. Sandborn WJ, Loftus EV (2004) Balancing the risks and benefits of infliximab in the treatment of inflammatory bowel disease. Gut 53(6):780–782
100. Dixon WG et al (2010) Influence of anti-tumor necrosis factor therapy on cancer incidence in patients with rheumatoid arthritis who have had a prior malignancy: results from the British Society for Rheumatology Biologics Register. Arthritis Care Res (Hoboken) 62(6):755–763
101. Karran P, Attard N (2008) Thiopurines in current medical practice: molecular mechanisms and contributions to therapy-related cancer. Nat Rev Cancer 8(1):24–36
102. Vivarelli M et al (2008) Liver transplantation for hepatocellular carcinoma under calcineurin inhibitors: reassessment of risk factors for tumor recurrence. Ann Surg 248(5):857–862
103. Askling J et al (2011) Cancer risk with tumor necrosis factor alpha (TNF) inhibitors: meta-analysis of randomized controlled trials of adalimumab, etanercept, and infliximab using patient level data. Pharmacoepidemiol Drug Saf 20(2):119–130
104. Sigler L, Jedd FL (1969) Adenocarcinoma of the ileostomy occurring after colectomy for ulcerative colitis: report of a case. Dis Colon Rectum 12(1):45–48
105. Cuesta MA, Donner R (1976) Adenocarcinoma arising at an ileostomy site: report of a case. Cancer 37(2):949–952
106. Stryker SJ (1983) Primary stomal adenocarcinoma. An unusual complication of ileostomy. Dis Colon Rectum 26(1):47–49
107. Roberts PL et al (1989) Adenocarcinoma arising in an ileostomy. Report of two cases and review of the literature. Arch Surg 124(4):497–499
108. Cox CL et al (1997) Development of invasive adenocarcinoma in a long-standing Kock continent ileostomy: report of a case. Dis Colon Rectum 40(4):500–503

109. Nilubol N et al (2007) Mucosal dysplasia in ileal pelvic pouches after restorative proctocolectomy. Dis Colon Rectum 50(6):825–831
110. Derikx LA et al (2014) Prior colorectal neoplasia is associated with increased risk of ileoanal pouch neoplasia in patients with inflammatory bowel disease. Gastroenterology 146 (1):119–128, e1
111. Knupper N et al (2006) Adenocarcinoma of the ileoanal pouch for ulcerative colitis--a complication of severe chronic atrophic pouchitis? Int J Color Dis 21(5):478–482
112. Branco BC et al (2009) Adenocarcinoma following ileal pouch-anal anastomosis for ulcerative colitis: review of 26 cases. Inflamm Bowel Dis 15(2):295–299
113. Giebel GD, Sabiers H (1996) Ileal pouch-anal anastomosis for ulcerative colitis and polyposis coli: is the risk of carcinoma formation conclusively averted? Eur J Surg Oncol 22 (4):372–376
114. Heuschen UA et al (2001) Adenocarcinoma in the ileal pouch: late risk of cancer after restorative proctocolectomy. Int J Color Dis 16(2):126–130
115. Herfarth C, Heuschen G, Heuschen UA (1998) Malignant transformation in ulcerative colitis and surgical implications. Chirurg 69(10):1020–1027
116. Lofberg R et al (1991) Dysplasia and DNA aneuploidy in a pelvic pouch. Report of a case. Dis Colon Rectum 34(3):280–283; discussion 283–4
117. Veress B et al (1995) Long-term histomorphological surveillance of the pelvic ileal pouch: dysplasia develops in a subgroup of patients. Gastroenterology 109(4):1090–1097
118. Carey PD et al (1993) Primary adenocarcinoma in an ileostomy: a late complication of surgery for ulcerative colitis. Surgery 113(6):712–715
119. Imam MH et al (2014) Neoplasia in the ileoanal pouch following colectomy in patients with ulcerative colitis and primary sclerosing cholangitis. J Crohns Colitis 8(10):1294–1299
120. Kim BJ et al (2009) Trends of ulcerative colitis-associated colorectal cancer in Korea: A KASID study. J Gastroenterol Hepatol 24(4):667–671
121. Hughes RG et al (1978) The prognosis of carcinoma of the colon and rectum complicating ulcerative colitis. Surg Gynecol Obstet 146(1):46–48
122. Lavery IC et al (1982) Survival with carcinoma arising in mucosal ulcerative colitis. Ann Surg 195(4):508–512
123. Ritchie JK, Hawley PR, Lennard-Jones JE (1981) Prognosis of carcinoma in ulcerative colitis. Gut 22(9):752–755
124. Gorfine SR et al (2004) Restorative proctocolectomy for ulcerative colitis complicated by colorectal cancer. Dis Colon Rectum 47(8):1377–1385
125. Delaunoit T et al (2006) Colorectal cancer prognosis among patients with inflammatory bowel disease. Clin Gastroenterol Hepatol 4(3):335–342
126. Heimann TM et al (1992) Colorectal carcinoma associated with ulcerative colitis: a study of prognostic indicators. Am J Surg 164(1):13–17
127. Kavanagh DO et al (2014) Management of colorectal cancer in patients with inflammatory bowel disease. Tech Coloproctol 18(1):23–28
128. Watanabe T et al (2011) Ulcerative colitis-associated colorectal cancer shows a poorer survival than sporadic colorectal cancer: a nationwide Japanese study. Inflamm Bowel Dis 17(3):802–808
129. Jensen AB et al (2006) Survival after colorectal cancer in patients with ulcerative colitis: a nationwide population-based Danish study. Am J Gastroenterol 101(6):1283–1287
130. Larsen M et al (2007) Survival after colorectal cancer in patients with Crohn's disease: A nationwide population-based Danish follow-up study. Am J Gastroenterol 102(1):163–167
131. Shu X et al (2011) Survival in cancer patients hospitalized for inflammatory bowel disease in Sweden. Inflamm Bowel Dis 17(3):816–822
132. Inoue Y et al (2014) Chemoradiotherapy followed by restorative proctocolectomy with partial intersphincteric resection for advanced rectal cancer associated with ulcerative colitis: report of a case. Surg Today 44(2):387–390

133. Radice E et al (1998) Ileal pouch-anal anastomosis in patients with colorectal cancer: long-term functional and oncologic outcomes. Dis Colon Rectum 41(1):11–17
134. Wu XR et al (2013) Preoperative pelvic radiation increases the risk for ileal pouch failure in patients with colitis-associated colorectal cancer. J Crohns Colitis 7(10):e419–e426
135. Emami B et al (1991) Tolerance of normal tissue to therapeutic irradiation. Int J Radiat Oncol Biol Phys 21(1):109–122
136. Adenis A et al (2007) Bevacizumab and postponed suture leakages after surgery for ulcerative colitis and rectal cancer. Gut 56(5):734
137. Da Silva GM et al (2003) Histologic analysis of the irradiated anal sphincter. Dis Colon Rectum 46(11):1492–1497
138. Lorenzi B et al (2012) Short-term effects of neoadjuvant chemoradiotherapy on internal anal sphincter function: a human in vitro study. Dis Colon Rectum 55(4):465–472
139. Ito M et al (2009) Analysis of clinical factors associated with anal function after intersphincteric resection for very low rectal cancer. Dis Colon Rectum 52(1):64–70
140. Rodriguez-Enriquez S et al (2014) Canonical and new generation anticancer drugs also target energy metabolism. Arch Toxicol 88(7):1327–1350
141. Inoue Y, Kusunoki M (2010) Resection of rectal cancer: a historical review. Surg Today 40 (6):501–506
142. Inoue Y et al (2011) Push-back technique facilitates ultra-low anterior resection without nerve injury in total mesorectal excision for rectal cancer. Dig Surg 28(4):239–244
143. Kusunoki M et al (1992) Modified anoabdominal rectal resection and colonic J-pouch anal anastomosis for lower rectal carcinoma: preliminary report. Surgery 112(5):876–883

Chapter 7
Surgical Treatment for Colorectal Cancer in Crohn's Disease

Hiroki Ikeuchi, Motoi Uchino, Toshihiro Bando, Kei Hirose, Nobuyuki Hida, and Shiro Nakamura

Abstract Cancer associated with Crohn's disease (CD) has shown a recent increasing trend. However, early detection is difficult due to an absence of characteristic symptoms, and differentiation from CD-related symptoms is challenging. For effective surgical treatment, it is necessary to determine malignancy according to the type of lesions, such as small intestinal, colonic, and anorectal. Intestinal cancer is less frequent and difficult to reveal prior to surgery, as its final diagnosis is often made based on perioperative or postoperative pathological examination results. For colonic lesions, final diagnosis is obtained in a similar manner. Furthermore, outcome is reported to be poor, as most cases are progressing at the time of diagnosis.

It remains inconclusive whether patients with colonic cancer and CD with colonic dysplasia as a complication should be treated by segmental resection or total colectomy as in ulcerative colitis (UC) cases. The prognosis of cancer associated with anorectal lesions is poor, though some reports have suggested that it can be improved by preoperative chemoradictherapy. For cancer associated with anorectal lesions, rectal amputation is inevitable. However, for those cases with extensive lesions around the anus, sacroabdominal rectal amputation, for which the surgery is started from the anal side in the jackknife position and later changed to another posture, is frequently more advantageous than ordinary abdominoperineal rectal amputation. The important complication after rectal amputation is persistent perineal sinus (PPS). Vacuum-assisted closure (VAC) is sometimes performed but satisfactory results are yet to be reported.

Furthermore, it is important to establish a method of surveillance for early detection.

Keywords Crohn's disease • Surgical treatment • Colorectal cancer

---

H. Ikeuchi (✉) • M. Uchino • T. Bando • K. Hirose • N. Hida • S. Nakamura
Department of Inflammatory Bowel Disease, Hyogo College of Medicine, 1-1 Mukogawa-Cho, Nishinomiya, Hyogo 663-8501, Japan
e-mail: ikeuci2s@hyo-med.ac.jp

M. Kusunoki (ed.), *Colitis-Associated Cancer*, DOI 10.1007/978-4-431-55522-3_7

7.1 Introduction

The occurrence of cancer in CD was not appreciated until many years after the classic description of "regional enteritis" in 1932. Recently, it has been recognized that CD carries an increased risk for malignancy [1, 2]. Three types of gastrointestinal carcinomas occur more frequently in patients with CD than in the regular population: small bowel cancer, colorectal cancer, and carcinoma arising from perianal fistula [2–6]. The presence of anal carcinoma in CD is clearly associated with long-standing perianal fistula [7]. Especially, physicians should have a high level of suspicion of cancer in patients with long-standing perianal CD who have a change in symptoms.

Preoperative, operative, and postoperative care require expertise in CD and a concomitant knowledge of oncologic surgery.

7.2 Location of Cancer in CD

Operative procedures depend on the location of the tumor. It is said that the localization of a tumor differs geographically. When considering geographic variations, the risk of colorectal cancer associated with CD is significantly higher in North America and the United Kingdom in comparison to Scandinavian countries [8]. These results may represent the genetic, dietary, or environmental differences between the countries. Stahl et al. found in their series that only 17 % ($n = 4$) of cancers in CD patients were located to the rectum which was much lower than in sporadic cancer (38 %) [9]. On the other hand, 59 % ($n = 14$) were located to the ascending and transverse colon in the CD patients which was significantly higher than in sporadic cancer (28 %). Kersting et al. reported previous studies that showed that 39–50 % of CD-associated tumors are located in the rectum [5, 10–12]. In their study, the majority of CD-associated tumors were located in a segment of the intestine that was easily accessible to endoscopic examination.

On the other hand, Mizushima et al. reported that based on the fact 34 of 44 colorectal cancers (77.3 %) in Japanese patients with CD arose in the sigmoid colon, rectum, and anal canal/fistula [13]. There may be genetic and environmental factors associated with developing colorectal cancer in patients with CD. Table 7.1 shows the location of cancer in our CD patients. Twenty-two of 32 (68.8 %) patients are located with anorectal lesions.

Table 7.1 Location of cancer

Location	No.
Fistula	4
Enteroenteric	3
Enterocutaneous	1
Intestinal tract	28
Ileum	2
Cecum	2
Descending colon	1
Sigmoid colon	1
Rectum	6
Anal canal	8
Anal fistula	8

7.3 Preoperative Preparation

7.3.1 Specific Medical Problems

Anemia, hyperglycemia, and electrolyte abnormalities should be discovered and remedied prior to operation.

7.3.2 Stoma Site Marking

In a patient with rectal amputation, consultation with an enterostomal therapist should be made to assist in the placement of the proposed stoma. Ideally the site should be located over the rectus muscle on a flat area from deep skin folds and bony prominences. The surface of the abdomen should be evaluated in the supine, sitting, and standing positions as this will often demonstrate skin folds and creases not evident in the other position. Finally, the patient's belt line is determined and every effort is made to place the stoma below it.

7.3.3 Preoperative Antibiotics

Intravenous prophylactic antibiotics should be administered 1 h prior to surgery so that maximal tissue antibiotic levels are achieved at the time of the skin incision.

7.4 Preoperative Examination

The presence of a complex fistula, an associated stricture, and perineal pain prevents a thorough examination of the anus and perineal areas, thus making diagnosis of a concomitant carcinoma difficult. Devon et al. reported that 14 patients who complicated cancer of anus all had multiple imaging studies, including magnetic resonance imaging (MRI), CT, and endorectal ultrasound, but none of these studies were diagnostic of carcinoma [14]. The diagnosis of cancer was made preoperatively in 10 of 14 patients, usually after multiple biopsies. In four patients, despite multiple tissue biopsies, the diagnosis was made intraoperatively ($n = 2$) or postoperatively ($n = 2$) [14].

The outcome is the same as in sporadic cancer at a corresponding stage; however, the prognosis is often poor due to the advanced stage at diagnosis. There are no formal guidelines for screening and surveillance of cancers associated with CD in the lower rectum and perianal regions. Friedman reported that if the endoscopist is unable to pass the stricture and perform surveillance with a standard pediatric endoscope, a barium enema or CT colonography should be considered to evaluate the proximal colon, with possible referral to an expert center [15].

7.4.1 MRI Examination

For anorectal cancer, pelvic MRI is the best method for examining cancer localization and invasion, as well as its positional relationship with surrounding organs. An anal fistula carcinoma related to mucinous cancer frequently forms mucus retention; thus multilocular cyst-like findings are frequently observed in T2-weighted MRI images. Figure 7.1 shows T2-weighted MRI findings of a mucinous cancer case, with multilocular cysts indicated by an arrow.

7.4.2 FDG-PET Examination

Some recent reports indicated the potential of FDG-PET to assess CD activity [16–18]. On the other hand, there is no report of the potential of FGD-PET to assess CD-associated malignant tumors. In our study, we performed FDG-PET with four patients prior to the operation, and the results indicated that two were positive and two were negative. Based on our limited experience, the accuracy rate for FDG-PET is not high, possibly because of the high rate of mucinous cell-type carcinoma in CD-associated cancer. In addition, Whiteford et al. reported that the sensitivity of FDG-PET for detecting mucinous carcinoma was lower than that for nonmucinous cancer [19].

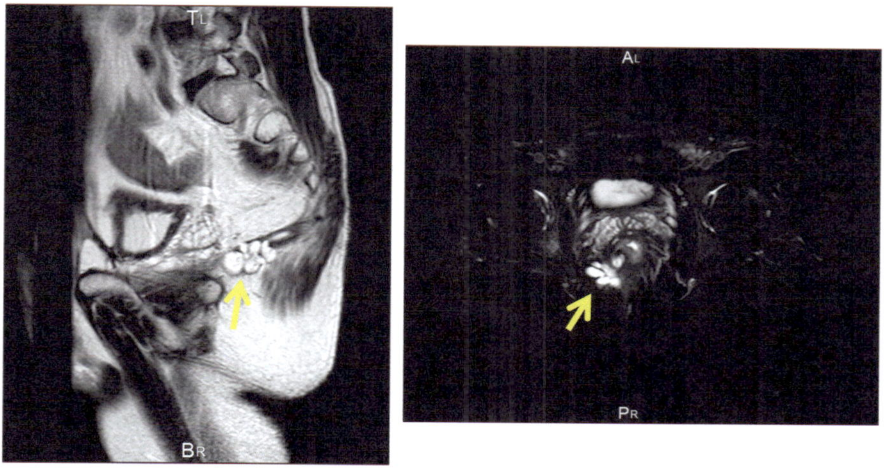

Fig. 7.1 T2-weighted images in patient with mucinous carcinoma. Multilocular cysts indicated by an arrow

7.4.3 *Curettage of the Fistulous Tract*

Severe chronic complicated perianal disease in patients who have CD seems to be associated with an increased risk for cancer in the lower rectum and anal canal. Laurent et al. noted that a high degree of suspicion for carcinoma must be considered during a rectal examination under anesthesia with biopsy, curettage, or brushing of the fistulous tract recommended [20]. The case which performed curettage of the fistula under anesthesia is shown in Fig. 7.2. The outflow of mucus is shown from a primary lesion.

7.5 Preoperative Treatment

7.5.1 *Preoperative Chemoradiotherapy*

No conclusions can be drawn regarding the efficacy of adjuvant chemoradiation in CD patients with fistula-associated anal adenocarcinoma because of the small population analyzed and the retrospective nature of the present study. Mucinous rectal adenocarcinoma has been associated with a lower response to chemoradiation than nonmucinous rectal cancer [21–23]. Sengul et al. compared the outcome after preoperative chemoradiation in 16 patients with mucinous rectal cancer and 55 patients with nonmucinous rectal cancer. Patients with mucinous tumors were found to have significantly more advanced T stages after chemoradiotherapy. Only

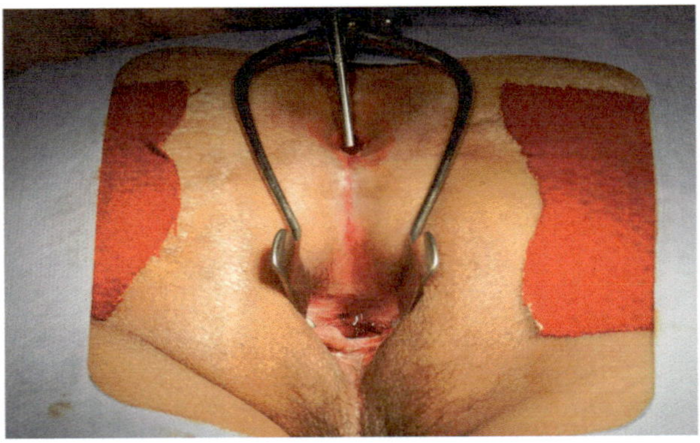

Fig. 7.2 Curettage of the fistula under anesthesia. This patient was diagnosed with mucinous adenocarcinoma

18 % of patients with mucinous cancer compared to 74 % of patients with nonmucinous cancer had a shift toward earlier T and N stages [21].

On the other hand, Wolfgang et al. reported that they had good results with combined neoadjuvant chemoradiation; all seven of their patients who received this treatment had a complete response, and they believe that neoadjuvant chemoradiation may play an important role in the treatment of locally advanced disease [24].

7.5.2 Case Presentation

Figure 7.3 shows the CD patients with complicated lower rectal carcinoma. He was 31 years old, and he had 15 years CD history. His preoperative pathological diagnosis was mucinous carcinoma. He was performed preoperative chemoradiotherapy and performed abdominoperineal rectal resection. Details regarding the per-treatment MRI examination, postoperative resected specimen, and pathological examination for that patient are provided in Fig. 7.3. He subsists without local recurrence 6 years after the operation.

7.6 Surgical Treatment

The objective of surgery for cancer in CD is resection of the cancer for cure or, when indicated, palliation and removal of associated or discontinuous segments of inflammatory disease when necessary. Surgical resection is generally accepted as the basic step in the treatment of these patients. Information on the adjuvant role of chemotherapy or radiotherapy is limited. Advanced rectal carcinomas are usually treated with preoperative pelvic irradiation. In patients with inflammatory bowel

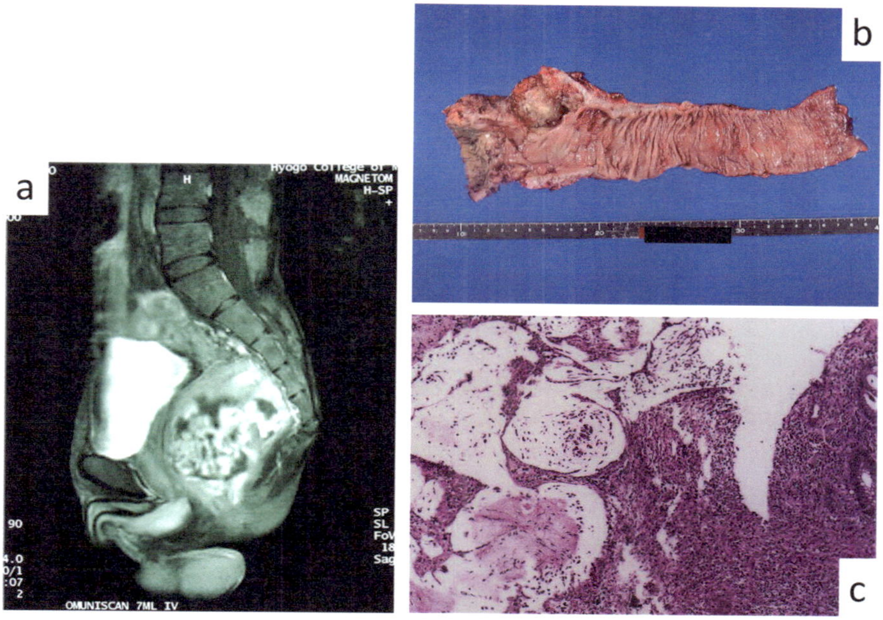

Fig. 7.3 CD-associated lower rectal carcinoma. (**a**) Preoperative MRI examination showing a tumor occupying most of the pelvic cavity. (**b**) Necrotic tumor specimen resected from the lower rectum. (**c**) Pathological examination results of a mucinous tumor with inflammatory cells. No malignant cells were found in this specimen

disease, however, this treatment produces an increased risk for severe gastrointestinal complications [25].

7.6.1 *Small Bowel Cancer*

7.6.1.1 Characteristic

There is a strong association between CD and small bowel cancer. The increased relative risk of small bowel cancer has been reported to be between 15.6 and 114.5 in comparison to the general population [26–30]. Cancer of the small intestine occurring in combination with CD is not as common as cancer of the large intestine. In addition, since cancer of the small intestine developing in patients with CD occurs in infected regions, it is very difficult to detect the disease at an early stage. This is because X-ray images of small intestinal cancer are similar to the images of strictures in patients with CD.

Making a definitive diagnosis of combined cancer was not possible before surgery, and the definitive diagnosis is obtained based on an intraoperative or postoperative pathological diagnosis. Palascak et al. reported that small bowel cancer was difficult to diagnose and was made preoperatively in only 1 of 20 patients who had CD as compared with 22 of 40 patients who had sporadic adenocarcinoma [31].

If we encounter such cases, we worry about whether to perform the reoperation or not, because the basic of surgery differs from CD and cancer.

7.6.1.2 Operative Procedure

Segmental resection is the performed surgical therapy for small bowel cancer in segmental CD. In patients with multiple small bowel strictures, concomitant strictureplasties should be performed in addition to the resection of the malignant stricture. Each stricture should be biopsied with frozen section evaluation to rule out the presence of synchronous cancers before a strictureplasty is carried out [32].

7.6.1.3 Case Presentation

A male developed diarrhea and fever at the age of 18 years and was diagnosed with CD in a detailed investigation. He had poor compliance to the prescribed drug therapy and visited the hospital on an irregular schedule. At the age of 34, he was admitted to our hospital for close examination of repeated ileus symptoms that had begun about 4 months prior to treatment. As the ileus symptoms became aggravated, a long tube was inserted. Figure 7.4 shows findings obtained in a series of images of the small bowel, in which a lesion suggestive of internal fistula was noted near the terminal ileum.

Surgery was performed to remove the segment. During the laparotomy, multiple nodes were found in the peritoneal cavity and subjected to an intraoperative pathologic examination, which led to a diagnosis of peritoneal dissemination of a poorly differentiated adenocarcinoma. The lesion was surgically removed and an artificial anus was created on the opening side. The resected specimen is shown in Fig. 7.5. Cancer invasion was observed up to the serous surface and distention of the

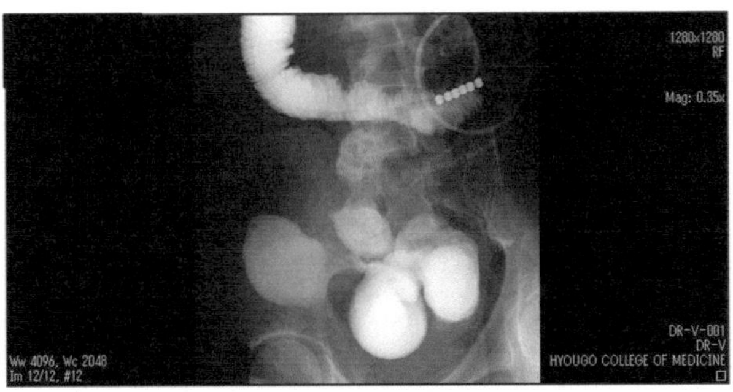

Fig. 7.4 Preoperative small intestinal examination

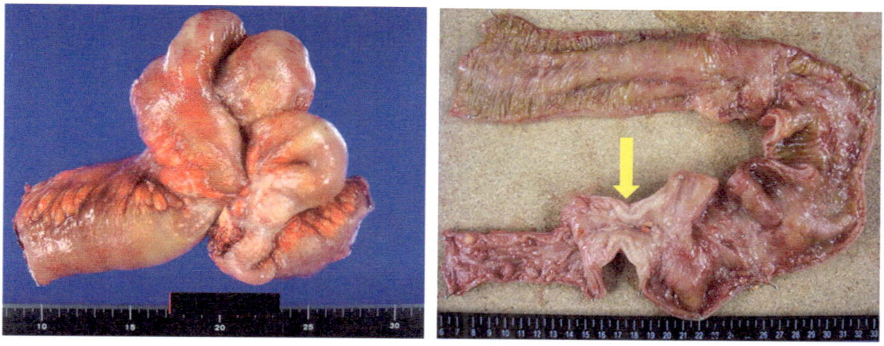

Fig. 7.5 Resected specimen in CD patient with small intestinal cancer. A lesion suggestive of internal fistulation was noted near the terminal ileum

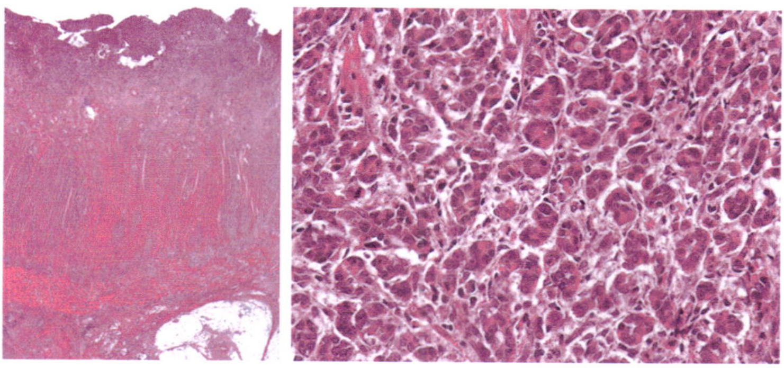

Fig. 7.6 Postoperative pathological findings. We determined that this was a case of poorly differentiated adenocarcinoma

gut on the opening side. We determined that this was a case of poorly differentiated adenocarcinoma (Fig. 7.6).

7.6.2 Colon Cancer

7.6.2.1 Segmental Resection

Segmental resection is the performed surgical therapy for colonic cancer in segmental CD.

7.6.2.2 Subtotal Colectomy

Subtotal colectomy is the procedure of choice in the presence of CD of the colon with malignant degeneration and sparing of the rectum. Following an abdominal colectomy, long-term surveillance with yearly endoscopy and biopsies of the remaining rectal segment is essential.

7.6.2.2.1 Case Presentation

A 30-year-old woman underwent complete resection of the colon and an ileostomy for multiple colonic lesions and a rectovaginal fistula. Thereafter, there was no close examination of the rectum as no aggravation of the rectovaginal fistula was noted. During a uterus cancer screening examination at the age of 40, an adenocarcinoma was found. She then came to our hospital for careful investigation of the remaining rectum, in which a carcinoma was found in a rectovaginal fistula on the rectal side. She underwent amputation of the remaining rectum. The resected specimen is shown in Fig. 7.7.

7.6.2.3 Total Proctocolectomy (TPC)

This procedure is generally performed for colonic cancer patients with pancolitis or with segmental colon and rectal disease or with colon and severe perianal disease.

7.6.2.4 The Surgical Treatment of CD-Associated Dysplasia

It remains unresolved whether total proctocolectomy is required for colorectal cancer or dysplasia in CD as it is in UC or whether segmental resection might be adequate [33]. In CD, once dysplasia is identified, segmental resection is a more feasible option, especially if there has been a consistent lack of inflammation elsewhere in the intestinal tract [33]. In the patients with multifocal colonic

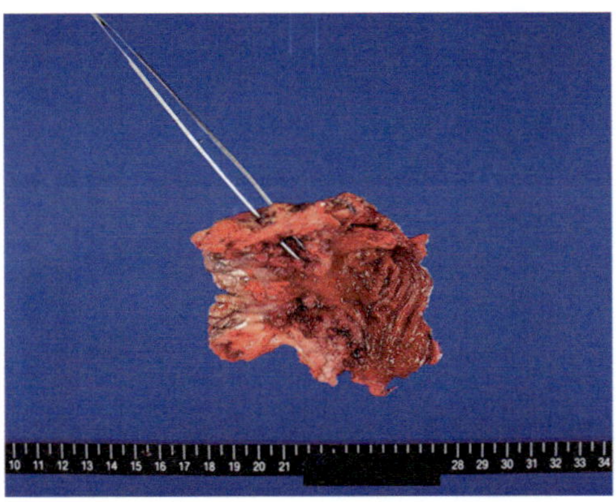

Fig. 7.7 Carcinoma in a rectovaginal fistula in a patient with CD

dysplasia or rectal dysplasia, the need for an aggressive approach, namely, TPC, is easily justified. Moreover, in CD patients with severe perianal disease or incontinence, TPC with end ileostomy offers treatment of the anal disability not provided by lesser resections such as segmental colectomy or IRA. Most surgeons favor TPC when cancer or dysplasia is discovered in the colon, but this usually results in a permanent ileostomy. Both total colectomy with ileorectal anastomosis (IRA) and segmental colectomy in CD patients with comorbidities are possible alternatives but require careful preoperative patient counseling regarding cancer risk and compulsive postoperative surveillance of any remaining colorectum.

There has been a case of colonic high-grade dysplasia (HGD) reported in a patient with CD that recurred as metastatic cancer despite subtotal colectomy followed by annual colonoscopy surveillance with biopsy [34]. Therefore, to make a definitive recommendation about the management of colonic dysplasia in CD, a large study would be required.

7.6.3 Cancer in Enteroenteric or Enterocutaneous Fistula

7.6.3.1 Characteristic

Cancer of the internal or external fistula occurring in combination with CD is not as common as cancer of the large intestine. In addition, it is very difficult to detect the disease at an early stage. This is because X-ray images of fistula cancer are similar to the images of usual CD patients.

The association between cancer and fistula has long been recognized [35–38]. Unfortunately such cancers are often unresectable. However, it is possible on occasion to carry out a radical "en bloc" resection including the fistula.

7.6.3.2 Case Presentation (Internal Fistula)

An ileal bladder fistula was found at around the age of 40 years old in a male patient, and surgical treatment was recommended. However, it was left untreated, as no symptomatic aggravation occurred. After hematuria continued for 1 month, he visited the urology department at the age of 54. A cystoscopic examination found a tumor, which was diagnosed as mucinous cancer based on biopsy findings. Total pelvic exenteration was performed. A perioperative radiogram image and the excised specimen are shown in Fig. 7.8. The patient died of cancer at 8 months after the operation.

7.6.3.3 Case Presentation (External Fistula)

An external fistulation was found between the descending colon and the skin in a 32-year-old woman, who was later referred to our hospital for surgery, as the fistula

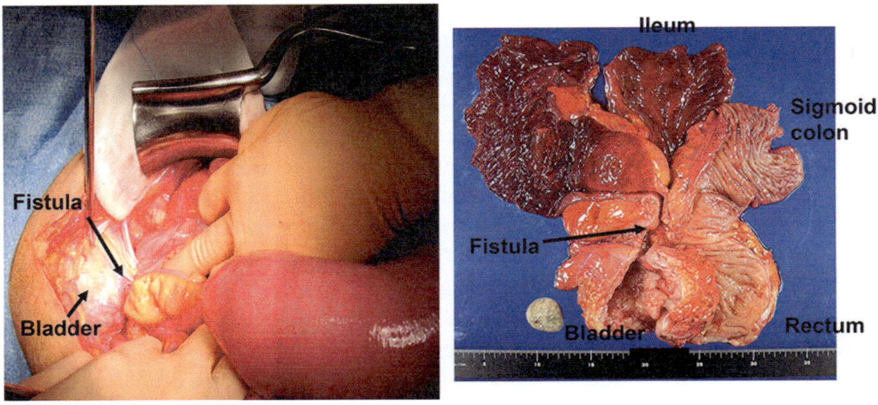

Fig. 7.8 Carcinoma between the ileum, sigmoid colon, and bladder in a patient with CD

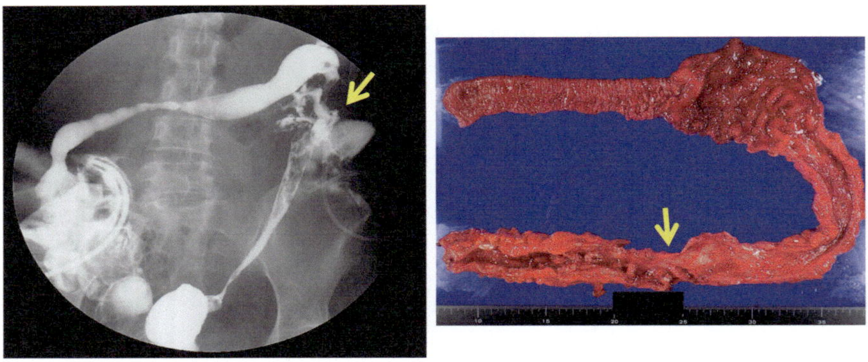

Fig. 7.9 Carcinoma between the descending colon and skin fistula in a patient with CD

did not close in spite of infliximab administration. Complete removal of the colon including 20 cm of the terminal ileum and an ileorectal anastomosis were performed. Preoperative contrast study and the excised specimen are shown in Fig. 7.9. In this case, cancer complication was demonstrated by a postoperative pathological examination of the specimen.

7.6.4 Anorectal Cancer

7.6.4.1 Characteristic

Severe chronic complicated perianal disease in patients who have CD seems to be associated with an increased risk for cancer in the lower rectum and anal canal.

Carcinoma arising in a chronic anorectal fistula in CD is rare, but the association has been reported in the literature. In most cases, it concerns a colloid carcinoma [25]. Probably chronic irritation at either end of a fistula can trigger the degeneration of scar tissue into cancer. The diagnosis is difficult, due to lack of specificity of symptoms and signs, and is often delayed, resulting in poor prognosis.

When considering prognosis, the degree of differentiation also known as the grade of the tumor is as important as the stage. Patients with well-differentiated tumors have a better prognosis and are less likely to require chemotherapy than those with poorly differentiated lesions. In CD, anal cancers more often are adenocarcinoma than squamous-cell carcinoma. Devon et al. reported that 14 of 3 patients had squamous-cell carcinomas, and the remainder had adenocarcinoma. Seven of the adenocarcinomas were well differentiated or moderately differentiated, and eight were of colloid or mucinous subtypes.

Mucinous adenocarcinoma usually occurs in about 10 % in sporadic colorectal cancer, but in cancer associated with CD, about 50 % have this more aggressive type of colorectal cancer [39].

On the other hand, Lee et al. reported that mucinous adenocarcinoma in a long-standing fistula in ano is known to be a slow-growing, locally aggressive neoplasm with a low-grade histologic appearance and rarity of metastasis. Tumor spread is usually lymphatic, and the inguinal lymph nodes are the most frequent sites of metastasis [40].

7.6.4.2 Operative Strategy

Treatment of rectal and anal cancer associated with CD involves proctectomy in the great majority of patients. In addition the colon should be resected or totally removed depending on the extension of the inflammation [41]. Treatment can be curative if the diagnosis is made early. The standard treatment option for these patients has been surgical. Abdominoperineal resection is the most frequently employed operation [42–44].

The mode of rectal amputation, i.e., abdominoperineal and sacroabdominal, is based on repositioning for the surgical approach. Ishigami et al. reported that intraoperative repositioning for patients undergoing rectal amputation helps reduce blood loss and operating time [45].

7.6.4.3 Case Presentation

Cancer that develops from a fistula around the anus is pathogenic for CD and requires extensive removal of the fistula. For surgery, sacroabdominal rectal amputation in a jackknife position is sometimes advantageous. Figure 7.10 shows a case in which an ileostomy and seton insertion were performed for aggravation of an ileal-anal lesion 10 years prior. The patient did not visit the hospital for that interim time period, as there were no symptoms, and then returned because of increased

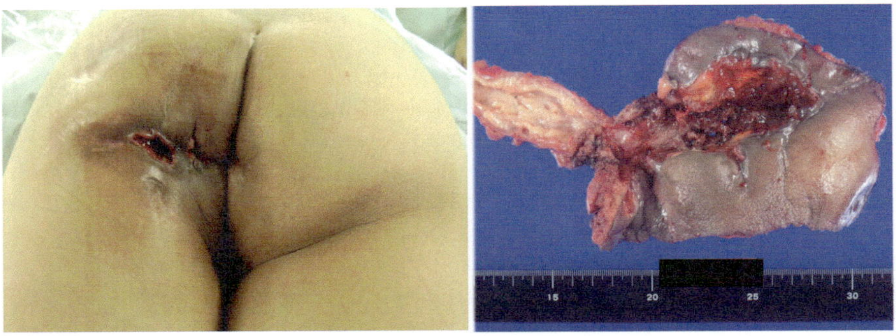

Fig. 7.10 Carcinoma in anal fistula in a patient with CD

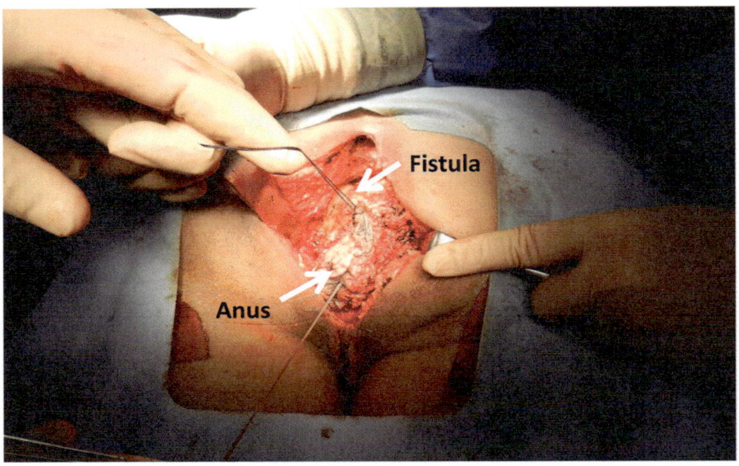

Fig. 7.11 Sacroabdominal rectal amputation

mucous excretion from the seton insertion site and pain. A pathological diagnosis of mucinous carcinoma was made. For surgery, a sacroabdominal rectal amputation was performed. Manipulation during rectal amputation on the anal side is shown in Fig. 7.11.

7.6.4.4 Pitfalls and Danger Points

Hurst reported that the abdominal perineal resection for CD entails potential pitfalls and danger points [46]. They include:

① Injury to autonomic nerves with resultant sexual and urinary dysfunction
② Ureteral injuries

③ Fecal contamination with resultant risk of intra-abdominal sepsis and wound infections
④ Improper plane of dissection along the sacrum resulting in excessive blood loss
⑤ Improper stoma placement and construction

7.6.4.5 Postoperative Complications

7.6.4.5.1 Perianal Wound Infection

Perineal wound infection often manifests with fever, perineal pain, and purulent drainage. When perineal wound infection occurs, the skin sutures are removed, and purulent fluid is completely drained. Perineal wound infection may result in a persistent perineal sinus.

7.6.4.5.2 Persistent Perineal Sinus (PPS)

Poor perineal wound healing after abdominoperineal resection for severe perianal CD was also reported by Marks et al. [47]. Persistent perineal sinus has been defined as a perineal wound that remains unhealed more than 6 months after surgery [48]. It was first reported in 1908 by Miles, as a complication of proctectomy, and it still occurs in an appreciable proportion of patients undergoing this kind of surgery [49]. Corman et al. studied 151 patients who underwent proctectomy for IBD and found poorer healing in those with CD than in those with UC [50]. In a more recent study of 427 similar patients, Bauer et al. reported primary healing in 95 % of patients with UC, but in only 67 % of those with CD [51]. Moreover, 13 % of patients with CD and only 0.8 % of those with UC had PPS after 6 months. Biopsy is recommended because chronic unhealed wounds may progress to carcinoma, especially squamous-cell carcinoma [52]. Successful management of the PPS depends on the clinical situation and the patient's condition. Conservative treatment and minor intervention, such as the application of a VAC device or curettage of the sinus, can be a feasible alternative to manage PPS.

Conservative Treatment

Conservative treatment of the sinus such as metronidazole ointment or fibrin glue can improve symptoms but often fails to achieve complete healing [52].

Vacuum-Assisted Closure

Vacuum-assisted closure (VAC) is a noninvasive, negative-pressure healing technique, which uses controlled subatmospheric pressure to remove excess wound fluid from the extravascular space, leading to improved local oxygenation and peripheral blood flow [53, 54]. There are several reports that VAC can accelerate perineal wound healing and promote the closure of cavities, as well as increase granulation and improve the adherence of a skin graft [52].

Surgical Treatment

A wide range of surgical techniques have been described to manage perineal wound problems depending on the patient's condition and the surgeon's preference. For details, please refer to the text book.

7.6.4.5.3 Urinary Retention

Postoperative urinary retention may result from intraoperative autonomic nerve injury. Urinary retention that resulted to autonomic nerve injury is best managed with intermittent catheterization. In most instances this is required for only a limited time as bladder function tends to recover. Long-term intermittent self-catheterization is rarely necessary [46].

7.6.4.5.4 Sexual Dysfunction

Impotence is an uncommon complication following total proctocolectomy and occurs in approximately 1–2 % of male patients [55]. Retrograde ejaculation, however, is more common and occurs in up to 5 % of males.

7.6.4.5.5 Stomal Complications

Complications related to the abdominal stoma are common and include peristomal fistula, peristomal hernia, and stricture. Up to 25 % of patients will require revision of their stoma to deal with one or more of these complications [56].

7.6.5 Palliative Procedure

When the cancer is very advanced or widely metastatic, surgical treatment may not offer any benefit to the patient. At times a palliative diverting stoma is all that may be performed or all that may be indicated.

7.6.5.1 Case Presentation

An intractable anal lesion was left untreated for a long period (Fig. 7.12). A biopsy was performed under anesthesia, which showed extensive mucinous cancer ranging

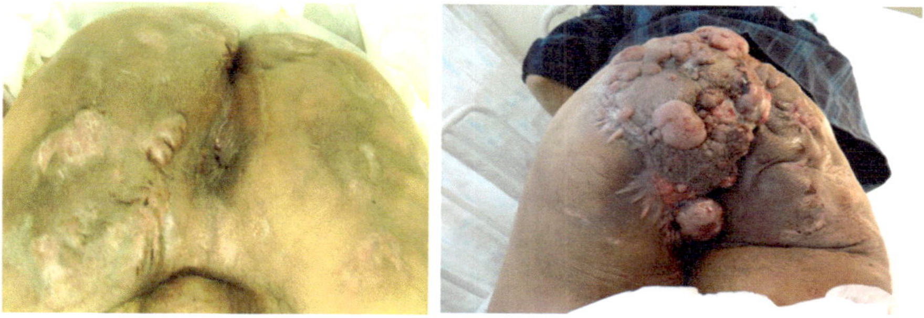

Fig. 7.12 Unresectable cancer case in a patient with CD

from around the anus to the femur, for which a radical operation was considered to be difficult (Fig. 7.12a). After a sigmoid colostomy, chemotherapy was started. The course was relatively favorable with successful local control for a period of 4 years. However, in postoperative year 5, the localized tumor became drastically enlarged and distal metastasis developed. The patient died of cancer at 5 years 10 months after surgery (Fig. 7.12b).

7.7 Postoperative Adjuvant Therapy

There is no data on the value and benefit of adjuvant therapy after curative resection of gastrointestinal cancers in CD. Recommendation for adjuvant therapy after resection of sporadic colorectal cancer can be adopted for the occasional patient with cancer complicating CD [32].

7.8 Postoperative Follow-Up

Following resection, long-term surveillance for the possibility of recurrence of the primary cancer by routine CEA or CA19-9 evaluation, as well as by CT or MRI examination when necessary, is reasonable recommendations.

References

1. Ullman TA (2003) Dysplasia and colorectal cancer in Crohn's disease. J Clin Gastroenterol 36:75–78
2. Sjödahl RI, Myrelid P, Söderholm JD (2003) Anal and rectal cancer in Crohn's disease. Color Dis 5:490–495

3. Jess T, Gamborg M, Matzen P et al (2005) Increased risk of intestinal cancer in Crohn's disease: a meta-analysis of population-based cohort studies. Am J Gastroenterol 100:2724–2729
4. Ky A, Sohn N, Weinstein MA et al (1998) Carcinoma arising anorectal fistulas of Crohn's disease. Dis Colon Rectum 41:992–996
5. Connel WR, Sheffield JP, Kamm MA et al (1994) Lower gastrointestinal malignancy in Crohn's disease. Gut 35:347–352
6. Higashi D, Futami K, Kawahara K et al (2007) Study of colorectal cancer with Crohn's disease. Anticancer Res 27:3771–3774
7. Lesalnieks L, Gaertner WB, Glaβ H et al (2010) Fistula-associated anal adenocarcinoma in Crohn's disease. Inflamm Bowel Dis 16:1643–1648
8. Canavan C, Abrams KR, Mayberry J (2006) Meta-analysis colorectal and small bowel cancer risk in patients with Crohn's disease. Aliment Pharmacol 23:1097–1104
9. Stahl TJ, Schoetz DJ, Roberts PL et al (1992) Crohn's disease and carcinoma: Increasing justification for surveillance? Dis Colon Rectum 35:850–856
10. Kersting S, Bruewer M, Laukoetter MG et al (2007) Intestinal cancer in patients with Crohn's disease. Int J Color Dis 22:411–417
11. Nikias G, Eisner T, Katz S et al (1995) Crohn's disease and colorectal carcinoma: rectal cancer complicating longstanding active perianal disease. Am J Gastroenterol 90:216–219
12. Savoca PE, Ballantyne GH, Cahow CE (1990) Gastrointestinal malignancies in Crohn's disease. A 20-year experience. Dis Colon Rectum 33:7–11
13. Mizushima T, Ohno Y, Nakajima K et al (2010) Malignancy in Crohn's disease and clinical characteristics in Japan. Digestion 81:265–270
14. Devon KM, Brown CJ, Burnstein M et al (2009) Cancer of the anus complicating perianal Crohn's disease. Dis Colon Rectum 52:211–216
15. Freidman S (2006) Cancer in Crohn's disease. Gastroenterol Clin N Am 35:621–639
16. Neurath MF, Vehling D, Schunk K et al (2002) Noninvasive assessment of Crohn's disease activity: A comparison of ^{18}F-fluorodeoxyglucose positron emission tomography, hydromagnetic resonance imaging, and granulocyte scintigraphy with labeled antibodies. Am J Gastroenterol 97:1978–1985
17. Lemberg DA, Isseman RM, Cawdron R et al (2005) Positron emission tomography in investigation of pediatric inflammatory bowel disease. Inflamm Bowel Dis 11:733–738
18. Löffler M, Weckesser M, Franzius C et al (2006) High diagnostic value of ^{18}F-FDG-PET in pediatric patients with chronic inflammatory bowel disease. Ann NY Acad Sci 1072:379–385
19. Whiteford MH, Whiteford HM, Yee LF et al (2000) Usefulness of FDG-PET scan in the assessment suspected metastatic or recurrent adenocarcinoma of the colon and rectum. Dis Colon Rectum 43:759–767
20. Laurent S, Barbeaux A, Detroz B et al (2005) Development of adenocarcinoma in chronic fistula in Crohn's disease. Acta Gastroenterol Belg 68:98–100
21. Sengul N, Wexner SD, Woodhouse S et al (2006) Effects of radiotherapy on different histopathological types of rectal carcinoma. Color Dis 8:283–288
22. Bosset JF, Calais G, Mineur L et al (2005) Enhanced tumorocidal effect of chemotherapy with preoperative radiotherapy for rectal cancer: preliminary results-EORTC 22921. J Clin Oncol 23:5620–5627
23. Grillo-Ruggieri F, Mantello G, Berardi R et al (2007) Mucinous rectal adenocarcinoma can be associated to tumor downstaging after preoperative chemoradiotherapy. Dis Colon Rectum 50:1594–1603
24. Gaertner WB, Hagerman GF, Finne CO et al (2008) Fistula-associated anal adenocarcinoma: Good results with aggressive therapy. Dis Colon Rectum 51:1061–1067
25. Devroe H, Coene L, Mortelmans JM et al (2005) Colloid carcinoma arising in an anorectal fistula in Crohn's disease: a case report. Acta Chir Belg 105:110–111
26. Greenstein AJ, Sachar DB, Smith H et al (1981) A comparison of cancer risk in Crohn's disease and ulcerative colitis. Cancer 48:2742–2745

27. Ekbom A, Helmick C, Zack M et al (1990) Increase risk of large-bowel cancer in Crohn's disease with colonic involvement. Lancet 336:357–359
28. Gillen CD, Andrews HA, Prior P et al (1994) Crohn's disease and colorectal cancer. Gut 35:651–655
29. Persson PG, Karlen P, Bernell O et al (1994) Crohn's disease and cancer: a population based cohort study. Gastroenterology 107:1675–1679
30. Gollop JH, Phillips SF, Melton LJ et al (1998) Epidemiologic aspects of Crohn's disease: a population based study in Olmsted county, Minnesota, 1943–1982. Gut 29:49–56
31. Palascak-Juif V, Bouvier AM, Cosnes J et al (2005) Small bowel adenocarcinoma in patients with Crohn's disease compared with small bowel adenocarcinoma de novo. Inflamm Bowel Dis 11:828–832
32. Greenstein AJ (1997) Cancer. In: Michelassi F, Milsom JW (eds) Operative strategies in inflammatory bowel disease. Springer, New York, pp 379–386
33. Connelly TM, Koltun WA (2013) The surgical treatment of inflammatory bowel disease-associated dysplasia. Expert Rev Gastroenterol Hapatol 7:307–321
34. Friedman S, Rubin PH, Bodian C et al (2008) Screening and surveillance colonoscopy in chronic Crohn's colitis: results of a surveillance program spanning 25 years. Clin Gastroenterol Hepatol 6:993–998
35. Greenstein AJ, Sachar D, Pucillo A et al (1985) Cancer in Crohn's disease after diversionary surgery: a report of seven carcinoma occurring in excluded bowel. Am J Surg 135:86–90
36. Greenstein AJ, Gennuso R, Sachar DB et al (1985) Extraintestinal cancers in inflammatory bowel disease. Cancer 56:2914–2921
37. Lighdale CJ, Sternberg SS, Posner G et al (1975) Carcinoma complicating Crohn's disease: report of seven cases and review of the literature. Am J Med 59:262–268
38. Church JM, Weakley FI, Fazio VW et al (1985) The relationship between fistulas in Crohn's disease and associated carcinoma. Report of four cases and review of the literature. Dis Colon Rectum 28:361–366
39. Hamilton SR (1985) Colorectal carcinoma in patients with Crohn's disease. Gastroenterology 89:398–407
40. Lee SH, Zucker M, Sato T (1981) Primary adenocarcinoma of an anal gland with secondary perianal fistulas. Hum Pathol 12:1034–1037
41. Sjödahl RI, Myrelid P, Söderholm JD (2002) Anal and rectal cancer in Crohn's disease. Color Dis 5:490–495
42. Basik M, Rodriguez-Bigas MA, Penetrante R et al (1995) Prognosis and recurrence patterns of anal adenocarcinoma. Am J Surg 169:233–237
43. Nelson RL, Prasad ML, Abcarian H (1985) Anal carcinoma presenting as a perirectal abscess or fistula. Arch Surg 120:632–635
44. Abel ME, Chiu YS, Russel TR (1993) Adenocarcinoma of the anal glands: results of a survey. Dis Colon Rectum 36:383–387
45. Ishigami S, Kitaguchi K, Sakikubo M et al (2008) The significance of intraoperative repositioning for the patients who undergoing rectal amputation –Comparison study of tow surgical techniques which are abdominoperineal and sacroabdominal rectal amputation. Jpn J Gastroenterol Surg 41:475–480
46. Hunt R (1997) Abdominal-perineal resection. In: Michelassi F, Milsom JW (eds) Operative strategies in inflammatory bowel disease. Springer, New York, pp 313–325
47. Marks CG, Riche JK, Lockhart-Mummery HE (1981) Anal fistulae in Crohn's disease. Br J Surg 68:525–527
48. Watta JM, Dombal RT, Goligher JC (1966) Long-term complications and prognosis following major surgery for ulcerative colitis. Br J Surg 53:1014–1023
49. Miles WE (1908) A method of performing abdominoperineal excision for carcinoma of the rectum and of the terminal portion of the pelvic colon. Lancet 2:1812–1913
50. Corman ML, Veidenheimer MC, Coller JA et al (1978) Perineal wound healing after proctectomy for inflammatory bowel disease. Dis Colon Rectum 21:155–159

51. Bauer JJ, Gelernt IM, Salk BA et al (1986) Proctectomy for inflammatory bowel disease. Am J Surg 151:157–162
52. Lohsiriwat V (2009) Persistent perineal sinus: incidence, pathogenesis, risk factors, and management. Surg Today 39:189–193
53. Yousaf M, Witherow A, Gardiner KR et al (2004) Use of vacuum-assisted closure for healing of a persistent perineal sinus following panproctocolectomy: report of a case. Dis Colon Rectum 47:1403–1407
54. Schaffzin DM, Douglas JM, Stahl TJ et al (2004) Vacuum-assisted closure of complex perineal wounds. Dis Colon Rectum 47:1745–1748
55. Bauer JJ, Gelernt IM, Salky B et al (1983) Sexual dysfunction following proctocolectomy for benign disease of the colon and rectum. Ann Surg 197:363–367
56. Post S, Herfarth C, Schumacher H et al (1995) Experience with ileostomy and colostomy in Crohn's disease. Br J Surg 82:1629–1633

MIX
Papier aus verantwortungsvollen Quellen
Paper from responsible sources
FSC® C105338

If you have any concerns about our products,
you can contact us on
ProductSafety@springernature.com

In case Publisher is established outside the EU,
the EU authorized representative is:
Springer Nature Customer Service Center GmbH
Europaplatz 3, 69115 Heidelberg, Germany

Printed by Libri Plureos GmbH
in Hamburg, Germany